Copyright 2006 by Dr. Judi Morris B.S.D.C

Foreword

The information contained in this book is not intended to be a substitute for professional medical advice, diagnosis or treatment of neck pain or neck injury. It is always wise to seek the advice of your doctor or other qualified health provider with any questions you have in regards to a medical condition. Never disregard professional medical advice or delay in getting help because of the content or the advice given in this book.

Preface

Just a little bit about me and why I am writing this book. Roughly fifteen years ago, I sustained an injury to my neck: two ruptured discs, torn and strained muscles, and a major tear in the sternocleidomastoid muscle (SCM). I was laid up for almost two years and not getting any better. There were lots of tests done, physical therapy, pain medication, muscle relaxants - the whole works! Many of you I am sure have been down this path as well. The medical doctors finally gave up, and told me I just had a bad neck. They gave me an endless supply of pain medication and sent me on my way. To me, that was a death sentence! I felt there had to be another solution. I eventually found my way to a chiropractor who helped me tremendously. Within three weeks my pain had diminished so much that ibuprofen was sufficient to control the pain. After a couple more months, I was off pain medication all together. This worked so well for me that decided to become a chiropractor myself. However, nothing can cure the damage that was done to my neck. Through this experience and working with my patients, I finally learned how exercising, stretching, and strengthening can prolong, and even help, muscles to heal and reshape to function better. I learned how to control my chronic pain. Thus, I have put together a program that has long lasting benefits!

Knowledge is a wonderful thing and in this book are tools that will help you, tools that are easy to learn but have a terrific impact on controlling your pain. Most of the program is designed to be incorporated in your daily activities and can be done as frequent as needed. Muscles when strengthened can be a powerful defense against pain, after all the muscles support the joints, help to protect them and allow us to move.

As a reminder...

Neck pain can sometimes be a very serious symptom. Be sure to check with your physician first before embarking on any exercises or at home remedies. You want to make sure all the nasty stuff has been ruled out first. Then if there are no tumors or serious disc problems, diseases etc...and your physician clears you to do your own exercises then continue to read on and find some tools to help you to lessen your pain and get control of your life again.

Table of Contents

Chapter 1

Understanding What Your Neck is...

I find that it helps to understand what your pain is all about. Frustration comes from hurting worse today then you did yesterday even though you didn't do anything for the pain to get worse. But that seems to be the nature of chronic pain. Some of us go around looking for a magic remedy that will instantly take away whatever is wrong so we can go back to the way we were. Unfortunately this is likely not going to happen. In many cases these things have a tendency to get worse with time instead of better. However, there is some good news... there are things that can be done to control the situation and to help you live a more normal and functional life, hopefully without medication. So, let's get started...from the beginning. Knowing what is in the neck and perhaps what may be causing your pain will help. It will also help to know how common injuries occur, what happens when we get older, and what we can do to help it from getting worse. Being healthy and taking a proactive stance in your health is one of the best things you can do for yourselves, but it is a lot of work and there is a lot of information out there that is often confusing and often doesn't seem to work. Through all the research that I have done, the people I have talked to, and my own experiences (and that of my patients), I have taken this knowledge and put together a program that gives you the tools to help yourself. Let me, once again, emphasis that taking care of yourself can be a lot of work and frustrating, and that makes it seem hopeless. But as you develop this program for yourself, and you practice and learn, I want you to look at your situation a year from now. It is my hope that you will discover that you are in fact better than you were a year ago. Changes can be subtle. We all have a tendency to forget how much or how bad the pain was. Your activity level will gradually increase, but you may not notice this until you think about it. For example, last year it took you two days to mow the lawn, and now you did it all in one day. Your pain and stamina have increased you just didn't notice!

Anatomy of a neck
Bone structure...

Let us begin our study with some basics of what the neck is and how it is put together. The neck function is to hold our head up, and in conjunction with the rest of the back, it is also a conduit for the spinal cord to travel through and distribute nerves to all parts of the body. These nerves sprout off of the spinal cord much like a tree sprouts branches. These branches travel through little holes in the vertebral column that are created by joints. Each nerve goes somewhere to innervate something, whether it is the heart, lungs, or a muscle to raise your arm to scratch your head.

The neck is formally known as the cervical spine. The cervical spine is made up of the first seven vertebrae (counting down from the head) of the spine. Your head literally sits on the top of the vertebrae known as the 'atlas'. The atlas was named after the Greek god who supported the weight of the world on his shoulders. Thus the weight of your head is supported by the atlas. The 2nd vertebra is known as the 'axis'. These two vertebrae work together to help you rotate your head from side to side. There are also special ligaments between the two vertebrae that allow for this rotation.

Figure 1.1

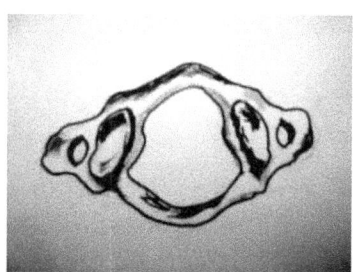

Atlas – C1

Axis – C2

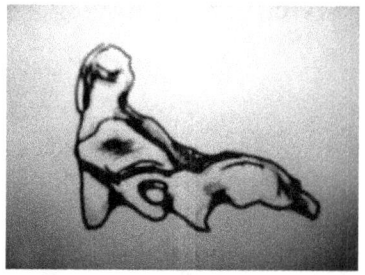

The dens fits up into the atlas and provides a fulcrum for pivoting the head. Note the kidney shaped areas on either side, this is the bottom half of the joint upon which your head sits.

Figure 1.2

C1 & C2 together from the side view. Note how the upper portion of C2 extends slightly above C1. As you can see this provides a fulcrum which to rotate.

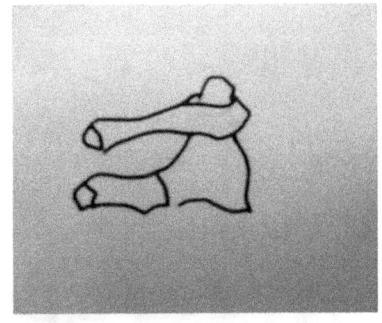

The remainder of the vertebrae in the neck helps you to bend your head forward and backward as well as to turn your head from side to side. Between each vertebrae are 'discs', these are made of special material that allows cushion between the vertebral bodies acting then as a sort of shock absorber. The discs in the neck, like the lower back, are thicker in the front which contributes to the normal curvature of these areas. In young adults the discs are strong, but as age progresses they are subject to degenerative changes becoming softer and weaker. Micro tears in the disc have been reported to occur as early as in the teenage years. Minor strains may cause damage and create unequal tension resulting in dysfunction of the joints. Unequal tension in the joint can cause muscle spasms. As a matter of course through various ways they may start to diminish in size or can become ruptured, this will allow problems to arise as we will discuss later. The whole of the vertebrae are then joined together by other ligaments that help to hold it together while you bend and twist around.

Figure 1.3 Cervical spine

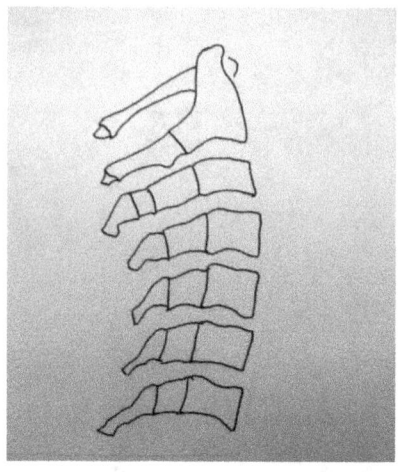

There are a total of seven vertebrae that make up the cervical spine. Each one is labeled as a number. In other words, the very top vertebra is C1, aka 'Atlas'. The very last vertebra is C7. This is a transitional vertebra because it is the last one before going into the upper back, or more commonly known as the Thoracic vertebrae. C5 and C6 is the stress level of the neck where most damage and injury occur.

In Figure 1.3 you will notice that this picture compromises the whole of the cervical spine, a side view. This view allows us to see the normal curvature of the spine as well as the disc spaces which are located between each of the vertebrae. To be a little more precise, the square portion of the vertebra is called the 'body'. Between each body of the vertebrae is where the discs are located. See Figure 1.5. If you'll remember the front portion of the disc is thicker, this helps to achieve a normal lordosis or curvature of the cervical spine. This normal curvature is commonly referred to as a 'C' curve. The normal 'C' curve of the neck can be important to help relieve pain and to allow for proper joint function. A loss of the curvature can prevent the motion of the neck from working correctly. When the neck is viewed from the front it should be vertical, straight up and down. If a curvature occurs from this view, it is sometimes termed scoliosis. At any rate an alteration in curvature from either view can put more stress upon the neck. Increased wear and tear may lead to joint dysfunction and pain.

In Figure 1.4, is a picture of the whole spine. There are five regions: cervical, thoracic, lumbar, sacral and coccyx. When all the regions are combined, notice the overall 'S' shape. Also note that each section has a 'C' curve. This is important in that this optimal curve allows for joints to function freely and easily. The 'S' shape helps to absorb any shock or jarring that occurs, such as when we jump or run or even with walking there is a certain amount of G-force that is produced, the 'S' shape helps to absorb that shock. Promoting this 'S' curve in yourself will also help to reduce pain, as it allows the joints to function without sustaining a constant jarring. Because of the many joints between each two vertebrae, a constant jarring can disrupt the integrity of the joint, especially in view of such factors as the disc weakening with age. In some studies it has all ready been proven that as early as age 15 there are tiny cracks within the disc. Muscles can properly function with proper position and alignment of the bony structures and the joints. They will also have better strength and endurance to resist wear and tear, and use less energy than when the bony structures are misaligned.

Figure 1.4 – Whole spine

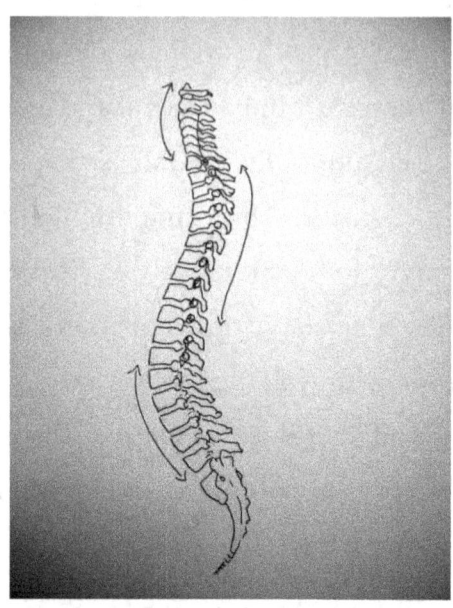

The top arrow represents the first region… Cervical spine, note also that the normal lordosis is a C shape. The next region is the Thoracic region or upper back. It too has a normal curve shaped as a C. The third region is the Lumbar or lower back, also C curved. Below the lumbar is the Sacral region followed by the Coccyx region at the very tip. When all the curves are combined you can see that an 'S' shape has occurred forming a large spring that helps to absorb shock such as when walking. At each heel strike when you walk, a G-force is sent up through the body. The 'S' shape helps to absorb this shock therefore offering some protection to your spine.

Joints

Structure and function...

If we look a little closer and take just two of the vertebra and examine them, we will find that there is a three-joint complex that is commonly called the facet joint. See Figure 1.5. These joints compromise the functional spinal unit, the facet joints and the intervertebral disc articulation (motion). The placement and angular degree of the facet joints in the cervical spine are what allows for the ranges of motion of the neck and help to create stability of the neck. There are two facet joints between each pair of vertebra, one on each side. This joint is classified as a synovial joint, or fluid filled joint, which allows the bones to glide with movement so friction is not created. The facet joint is also a source of pain when things go wrong such as disc disease, misalignment, arthritis, and a variety of other problems.

The two typical vertebras (Figure 1.5) show a facet joint. This is the area in the picture where the top vertebra and the bottom vertebra are touching. The vertebral body is the square most portion. In between these two vertebral bodies lays the disc.

Figure 1.5

Intervertebral foramen - where the nerves pass through

Facet Joint 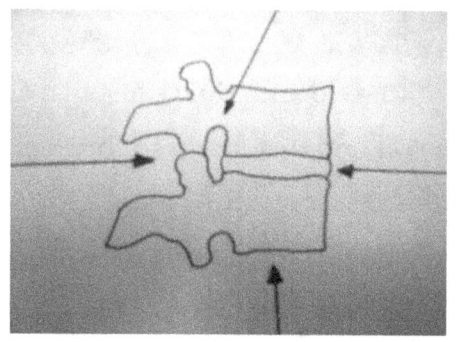 Disc

The Vertebral body

Figure 1.6

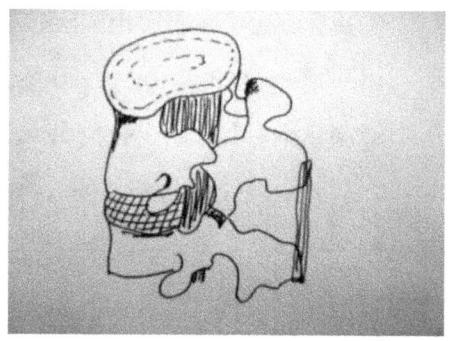

The picture (Figure 1.6) shows a view of two vertebras from an angle behind the body of the vertebra. Note the checkered portion is the area of the disc. The vertical lines directly behind the vertebral bodies indicate ligaments. The outer most portion of the vertebra, beyond the body, is the spinous processes and other structures. Although, from this view it is difficult to see, the area of the spinal cord itself is in the center, behind the vertebral body, but in front of the outer boniest structures that include the spinous process. The spinal cord is well protected by all the bony prominences.

The space that is created between the body of the vertebrae and the facet joint is termed the intervertebral foramen. In Figure 1.6 note the oval or kidney shaped space that is created when the facet of each vertebra join to form the facet joint. This creates an opening for the nerves and blood vessels to pass through. The spinal cord is contained in the posterior structure behind the vertebral body and coming out of the spinal cord. The peripheral nerves act like tree branches which pass through the intervertebral foramen and continue to branch out to the rest of the body. When tissues within the opening get inflamed or swell, it causes pressure on the nerves and can be a source of pain. When the pressure is coming from a disc it is often referred to as nerve impingement. This can produce sharp pain extending into the shoulder or down the arm, sometimes numbness and tingling may occur.

Just as a side note, the diagrams that have been shown are simplified to make understanding a little easier. The neck is very complex and many nerves can be pinched in someway or another. The disc itself has nerves that can also be pinched and are often an intrinsic source of pain. As aging occurs, the discs weaken and are more susceptible to injury, even to the point of rupture. The disc has a soft center that leaks out into the surrounding area, when this occurs it is sometimes called a rupture. This soft substance is caustic in that it can cause irritation to the tissue it encounters. If there is bulging of the disc, then the disc is compressed enough to overstretch its boundary. In either case this produces unwanted substance in the surrounding tissue and compromises available space, thus compressing other structures. This produces irritation to the structures all ready present and to the disc itself. As with any irritation if done long enough it will produce pain and often sets up a chain reaction into other structures surrounding the joint such as muscles. The intervertebral foramen is a common source of pain because of this encroachment into the allotted space either from the disc, soft tissues, inflamed nerves, or variety of things. Suffice it to say when this space is compromised pain is often the result.

Pain - What makes it happen...

Pain is defined as the unpleasant sensation which may be associated with actual, or potential, tissue damage. It is the body's way of telling you that something is wrong and you need to take action. As a result of tissue damage and during the healing process scar tissue is often formed. Most of the previous discussion has been on sources of irritation which produce pain. It would be correct to state that because of a dysfunction there is irritation which eventually produces pain. Chronic pain of which this book is about is usually of source of irritation from a dysfunctional unit. Get rid of the irritation, the pain is gone.

So far we have discussed some of the causes connected with what can produce irritation, such as joint dysfunction, misalignment of joint, swelling of tissues, encroachment, disc disease, and aging.

All of these can have the ability to produce pain and mostly likely can be one of the components of chronic pain.

The body is basically symmetrical, in that each side mimics the other side. The same is with the joints. The facet joint on each side, see Figure 1.5, when misaligned creates an asymmetry. The joints on opposite sides are not functioning together. This dysfunction can be caused by a series of events and/or disease such as disc disease, loss of normal curvature, etc. This in turn creates an asymmetry in the discs, muscles, ligaments, and tendons attached to the joint. Chronic joint dysfunction or misalignment can then create a source of constant irritation and resultant pain; therefore proper joint function becomes important. Because the discs do not have their own blood supply, (it should be noted that the discs receive their blood supply from the motioning of the joint) the disruption of proper joint function can cause disruption in the disc itself. The proper motioning of the joint allows the blood to flow in and out, thus essentially nourishing the disc. As the joint begins to malfunction then its source of nutrient, blood supply, becomes altered. A lack of proper blood supply will cause the disc then to shrink and dry out ultimately decreasing the size of the disc and therefore the opening through which the nerves pass through. This of course would cause further irritation to the surrounding tissues and once again be a source of pain. If the lack of blood supply is contained to one area within the disc, it can create a wedged appearance where one side is operating ok and the other side is 'crimped' creating a 'pinched' nerve effect, see Figure 1.7. Pinched nerves can also be caused by a swelling of the tissues either from inflammation or scarring of the tissues as a result of any inflammation.

Figure 1.7

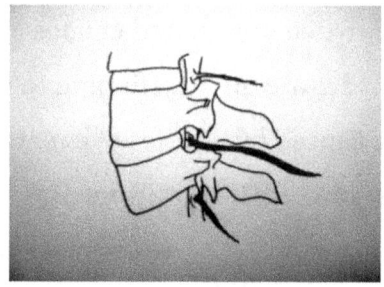

The dark strings are nerves coming through the intervertebral foramen. The middle one is 'pinched', note how much smaller the opening is when compared to the one above.

Figure 1.8

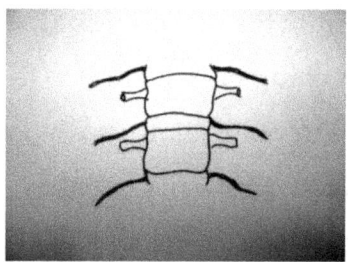

Remember the square portion is the vertebral body. Between each of the vertebral body is the disc. Then behind this is the spinal cord with the branches of nerves coming through each intervertebral foramen which is created when the facets join to each vertebra. Notice how the nerves (blackened string like projections) protrude out at approximately the same level as the disc.

Muscles - What happens...

There are many muscles attached as well that help move the neck, arms and head as well as the vertebral joints. The smaller muscles that actually surround the joint are important as they aide in protecting the joint and are important in maintaining posture. The larger muscles help to support the head and motion.

I need to mention some of the muscles that tend to develop trigger points and spasms. Trigger Points are tiny points in muscles that develop when a muscle has been injured or overworked. When they become irritated they send out pain signals often to a referring site. The first muscle of discussion is the SCM (sternocleidomastoid muscle) as you see in Figure 1.9 it runs along the side of your neck into the front. It helps you to tilt your head toward the same side of your shoulder, to tilt your head and neck downward, and raises your head up while you are lying down. The SCM is the one to blame for your 'stiff' neck. When it spasms, it can be very hurtful, limiting the movement of your neck while turning from side to side. Most often it is just the one side that is involved but an episode of stiffness can last for days.

The next large muscle that needs to be mentioned is the trapezius (Figure 1.9); a triangular shaped muscle that covers the upper back and neck. This muscle bends the head and neck backwards and towards your shoulder. It also is important in helping you maintain an erect shoulder posture. This muscle when irritated will make the top part of your shoulders ache and burn, especially when you have been sitting and working at your computer for a while or simply just reading with your head bent down.

Some of the smaller muscles of great importance in the neck are three of the muscles located on the side and front of your neck named the scalenus muscles. Actually there is a set on each side of your neck. (See Figure 1.10) The scalenus muscles are labeled anterior, medius, and posterior. The anterior scalenus helps rotate your neck to the opposite side, bend to the same side, and bends the neck forward. The medius and the posterior scalenus help bend your neck to the same side. These guys get achy, stiff and burn sometimes when bending your head. They can limit how far you can turn your head to see what's behind you. These muscles become tight and sore creating stiffness with movement.

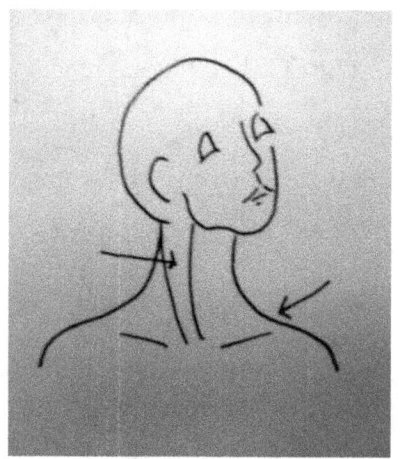

Figure 1.9

The left arrow is pointing to the SCM

The right arrow is pointing to the topside of theTrapezius.

The SCM muscle works to tilt your head to the shoulder, bending your head down and to raise your head up when you are lying down. This muscle is primarily involved with many 'stiff' necks. Trapezius muscle helps your head to bend and helps to keep shoulder position.

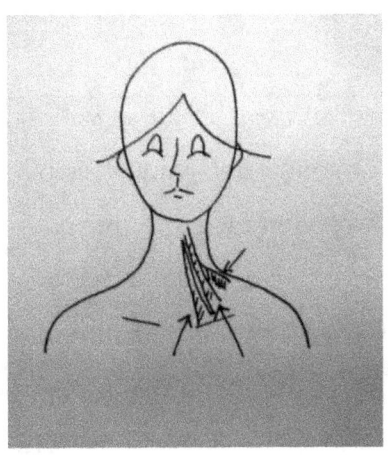

Figure 1.10

The top arrow is the posterior scalenus muscle; the middle area is the middle scalenus and the arrow to the left is the anterior scalenus. The other side of the neck has the same set of muscles, denoted as left or right. This group of muscles work hard to turn your neck and help it to bend side way and to bend downwards.

Figure 1.11

These two muscles are in the back of the neck, they extend down the neck from the back of the head and help to bend your head and neck backwards. They are from the semi spinalis group of muscles and tie directly into the vertebra.

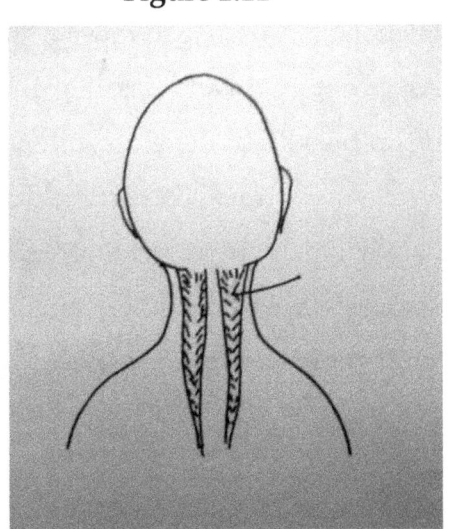

In the back of the neck are the semi spinalis capitis, Figure 1.11. This muscle helps to bend your head backwards, when they ache it feels hard to hold your head up.

Although there are many more muscles that haven't been named, these are some of the major players. All of the muscles work in synergist motion to perform actions such as bending, turning, twisting, raising arms and legs etc. They all are all important, but some of the time when one isn't working too well another can help to pick up the slack. As damage and injury occur the muscles may not work as well and can sometimes do funky things. One of those things is development of trigger points or to spasm. Motion of a healthy muscle is smooth and fluid. It should not be jerky and off kilter such as a damaged muscle may do. As part of rehabbing the muscles your job is to help make your muscles become more fluid and strong by practicing the exercises that follow and over time your actions will become smoother and more functional. A damaged muscle hurts; repairing that damage will reduce your pain and possibly give you more energy. Because of the problems that develop with posture and neck problems your muscles over time will become damaged as well, but strengthening them will help to protect the joints and the damaged area. It can all work together to get rid of pain or at the least reduce your pain. Put you in more control so to speak.

Chapter 2

Injuries - Background - How Injuries Occur

Neck pain, although not as common as back pain, can be just as debilitating. It can cause many people to alter their lifestyle and miss out on having a normal life. Missing out on enjoying what we like to do, even something so simple as trying to read a book or surf the internet. Today's traditional medicine offers muscle relaxants, pain medication, physical therapy, and surgery as tools to 'fix' the problem. As a Chiropractor I have, through many of my patients, found that often times these solutions are not the real answers. They offer a temporary patch that helps... at times, but the primary problem keeps recurring and often it gets worse. Over time it seems like many people make an unconscious, or a conscious, decision that there is no hope and they have to learn to live with their pain. Then in many subtle ways they begin to alter their lifestyles to avoid that pain. They stop playing basketball, stop going to the gym, stop running, stop swimming, stop mowing the yard, stop, stop, stop till after a while their tasks are limited to only what is necessary to make it through the day. They begin to count themselves lucky if they work all day, come home and can rest that evening without pain. However, most days there is pain, maybe not a lot, but its there, burning and aching.   A typical scenario might be...A man walks into the doctor's office with sudden neck pain, he says he woke up one morning with a stiff neck. Remember the SCM muscle? This happened two days ago and has been unrelenting since. What went wrong?

Without getting too technical or delving into much physiology, picture a canvas bag with a shoulder strap, if you never were to use the bag, the strap would stay intact and be 'healthy'. But if you load the bag with various things, books and what not, over time, the strap begins to fray. First one string then another till eventually the strap breaks and the bag is no longer functional. It's damaged. We can cut out the damaged area and sew what is left back onto the bag, but the area is still damaged and we have altered the biomechanics of the bag...permanently! We return to using our bag, just as we did before and again over time, the strap begins to fray and unless we alter the use of that bag, it will break again, only this time it doesn't take as long. The question then comes to mind, how can I continue to use the bag for what I need and not break the strap?

In the body, when imposed forces such as lifting and bending exceed the point of structural strength something always fails and that first string has frayed. While the same actions keep being performed, over time, the same thing keeps happening and we begin to experience that 'first' neck ache as more and more strings are frayed resulting in a breakdown of tissues. The minor 'neck ache' builds upon previous 'neck aches' till it becomes more frequent as we continue to do the same things. As the occurrences of neck aches continue, we begin to seek help. It maybe that first we ice the area; maybe we go to the store and get something off the shelf that helps to relieve the pain. There is plenty to choose from at the drug store, all offering temporary help. But, an important thing to remember is that pain alerts us that tissue damage has occurred. When the pain goes away scar tissue will have formed. With each neck ache, the scar tissue continues to build. Each episode of pain is causing tissue damage, resulting in a symptomatic breakdown of tissues, so that over time there is what is termed, 'chronic inflammation' of the site and chronic pain begins to develop.

When the pain gets bad enough, or occurs often enough, most people will seek professional help. Many people will go to a doctor of traditional values and receive pain medication, physical therapy, muscle relaxants, etc. The problem is that this only offers a temporary solution. This action will be repeated periodically when the pain becomes overwhelming. Muscle relaxants and pain medication will continue to mask the problem. As the inflamed area heals, more scar tissue is formed - more damage is done. Over time because of the frequent episodes of pain and stiffness, lifestyles are altered. Maybe if we put only two books in the bag, instead of four, the strap will not break. Maybe if we buy a lighter vacuum cleaner, maybe if we do not play football, maybe if we hire someone to do the yard work, get the kids to mow the lawn, have the neighbor shovel our snow, buy a snow blower, etc. A lot of people out there continue to suffer with pain silently; they may think there is nothing they can do.

In the neck, and through out the body, is a special type of tissue termed connective tissue. It has a specialized stretching ability that allows us to change positions. For example, sitting in a chair causes the tissue to stretch and bear the weight of our upper body on the tissue of the buttocks. As you might imagine the buttocks are flattened during our time of sitting, but when we stand up again it returns to its former shape. Because of its stretching ability it is particularly susceptible to overuse. For instance, a rubber band or a piece of elastic has a lot of the same properties of connective tissue, but when over stretched, or over loaded, it becomes permanently stretched or it breaks. Remember our canvas bag, due to overloading the bag, the strap eventually will start fraying at the edges, one fiber at a time. When we exceed the level of structural strength that we are capable of, our connective tissue becomes over stretched, resulting in injury, one fiber at a time. This is the underlying factor in most overuse and repetitive type injuries. A permanent deformation of the underlying tissue, which causes the joints to become unstable and more prone to repeated injury, commonly referred to as normal wear and tear. However, once a muscle is damaged it can be a great source of pain. Inflammation is one of the first processes that occur with any injury, the body will actually shorten the muscle as a way of protection when it becomes injured. This further complicates the dysfunction and instability of the joint.

We all have used an article of clothing that given enough time and wear the elastic looses its stretch and will no longer return to its original shape as when the article was new. The same can be said of our connective tissue. If we consider the point at where our canvas bag and the canvas strap join together as similar to a joint, we can begin to understand that over time with repetitive injury how the joint will weaken and become loosened or lax. This makes it much more susceptible to breaking apart. In the case of the canvas bag, we probably will find that we no longer put as much weight into it for fear of breaking on us, but in our bodies it is not so simple to see, thus we continue to overload.

Our bodies do have a backup or protective feature built in that will help to protect us from the instability of a loosened joint. When the joint has sustained enough injury and becomes unstable or loosened the body begins to compensate in many ways. Two of the most significant ways might be compensation of the muscles by over-development of the injured site and/or disc degeneration disease which appears to be the body's way of trying to stabilize the injured site.

In Figure 2.1 you will notice a rather simplified drawing of a muscle attachment to a bone. Notice that in the normal positioning the muscles are symmetric, meaning they are the same on each side of the bone. The point where two bones join together by ligaments, muscles and tendons is called a joint. On each side of the joint there is symmetry of the tissues attached to the joint.

Figure 2.1

The ligaments and tendons that attach the muscles to the bone are of very low blood supply and sometimes take up to a year to heal after an injury.

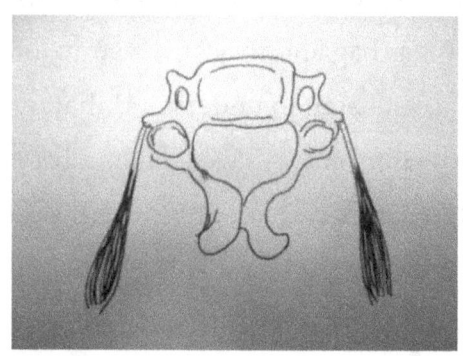

If after repetitive injury the joint becomes lax or loosened the joint then becomes unstable and can no longer do its job like it did before, so it compensates. In the next drawing, asymmetry has occurred by over-development of one side of the muscles.

Figure 2.2

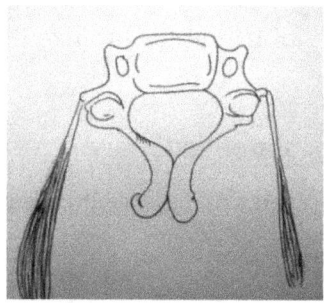

Often with an injured joint proprioreceptive fibers can become damaged as well. These fibers are responsible for contracting the muscle in response to a stimulus. A reduction in these important fibers can cause further future injuries, thus the need to stimulate their regrowth.

This asymmetry can often cause a domino affect within the body. For example, suppose that at C5 a minor injury has occurred, as in the case of any injury there will be:

1. A nerve component – research has shown that even a small amount of pressure on any spinal nerve can impact the function of the nerve

2. A muscle component – muscles are innervated by the nerves, they will also shorten protectively as a response to the injury

3. Soft tissue component – changes will occur to the surrounding ligaments, tendons, blood supply etc. as the nerve function is interrupted and the body responds to the injury

4. Chemical component – the body will send out certain chemicals in response to the injury to repair damage

5. The bone component - the vertebrae will be out of position or not moving in a coordinated fashion, instability will occur within the joint

Over a period of time this area will heal and the primary symptom of pain will have gone away. However looking more closely we see that there is a small amount of tissue damage that has resulted, and scar tissue has taken the place of normal connective tissue during the healing process. Now because a scar does not have the same stretching ability as normal tissue this area becomes more susceptible to repeated injury. Perhaps a week later or a month later, but most certainly at some point in the future this area will most likely be injured again. The same process then repeats itself; only this time as a result there is more scar tissue that has formed. With time and repeated injury the scar tissue builds, eventually the joint is no longer able to function at the same efficiency as it did without injury. The muscles, tendons and ligaments attached to the joint begin to remodel because of the joint malfunction and asymmetry develops. Since the adjacent structures also begin to malfunction because of overcompensation this eventually begins to affect the areas above and below the joint, before long the joints above and below C5 may begin to compensate their biomechanics (motion) because of C5. The Domino effect has begun and you may begin to notice that the frequency of your neck pain increases, the severity of the pain may also increase.

When a spinal joint is dysfunctional it creates instability within the spine, much like walking a tight rope the body will build spurs to help stabilize the joint just like you might stretch out your arms to steady yourself when walking a tight rope. If by building the spurs the spine is unable to steady itself, the spurring will continue to grow to the point it fuses the two vertebrae together. This whole process can occur very gradually, the episodic pain may have long intervals in between but it will almost always continue progressive deterioration. This condition is most often called Degenerative Disc Disease. While some books may argue that injury has nothing to do with it, that it is in fact just the aging process, I have found through my own studies that it occurs primarily as a result of repetitive injuries that accumulate over time. Thus resulting in joint instability, and the degeneration is the body's attempt to stabilize or adapt to improper healing of a previous injury.

Figure 2.3

Note the uneven edges on the vertebral body, the spurring and the loss of disc height.

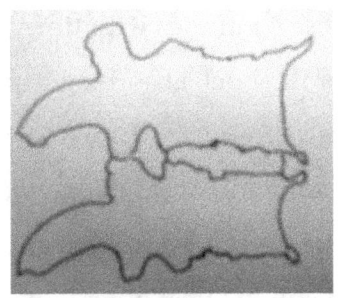

Degenerative Disc Disease and Degenerative Joint Disease are two terms that can be somewhat confusing. Degenerative diseases are thought to be just that - degenerative in nature, meaning that with time the breaking down process continues. So it would stand to reason in the case of Degenerative Disc Disease, the discs are degenerating. But why? A recent study shows that when a person has been in an automobile accident with a speed as little as 5mph, they will most likely develop Degenerative Disc Disease within ten years. Is it because they are ten years older? The assumption appears to be the effect of trauma.

What we do know is that the disc is a connective tissue and lacks a blood supply. We also know that the blood is fed to the disc by motion of the vertebrae above and below it. It would stand to reason that when motions of those two vertebras are disturbed then the disc are indirectly disturbed as well because their supply of nutrient is altered. So a better term then might be *abnormal* wear and tear as a result of many minor injuries that at the time might have been thought of as 'no damage done', I'm all right. After the first injury then successive injuries are easier to come by due to the weakened state of the joint. As the altered nutrient supply to the disc continues with time, the disc will begin to shrink and loose a lot of its shock absorbing capabilities, micro tears will occur making the disc itself more prone to injury, and collapse. Alteration of disc formation or function would then impact the overall mechanics of the two vertebras that support the disc. The damage then may begin to affect other joints of the vertebra, such as the facet joints perhaps causing arthritis to develop.

Facet joint pain is another source of pain that occurs in the neck and often is rather difficult to diagnosis, especially in the light of other problems in the neck. Generally speaking facet pain is often unpredictable and does not occur daily, but rather occurs frequently; and will probably be tender to touch. Typically the pain is more localized confining itself to the neck and shoulders. Arthritis may also be the source of the degeneration that is occurring in the facets. The symptoms are often presented with a complaint that when we use our neck more, the pain gets worse especially when bending the head backwards. As with any arthritis, inflammation is occurring in the facet joint because you are using it, and since the joint has nerve endings we feel that inflammation as pain. The irritation of the joint can also impact the muscles of the joint and cause spasms which will result in more pain and discomfort. The spasms really are just a protective mechanism by which your body is trying to help. A result of the pain is a tendency to stop motioning the neck, the more you use it the more you hurt, so you stop using it. But this lack of motion actually causes more problems and things will only get worse.

Although the jury is still out on the cause of arthritis, the end result is a dysfunctional joint that has periods of pain and swelling with periods of relative freedom. According to the Medline Medical Encyclopedia, of the arthritides, osteoarthritis is the most common, and is possibly related to injuries defined as the breakdown of cartilage allowing the bones to rub together and creating irritation, pain and inflammation. Note that osteoarthritis can occur at any age, but more often as we grow older. In theory then the older we get the more injury that has been sustained and therefore the more likely arthritis will occur.

Traditional treatment for arthritis is many of the non steroidal drugs such as Ibuprofen and the newer ones classed as Cox 2 Inhibitors, which are thought to be safer for long term use. The intent of these drugs is to reduce pain by inhibiting the inflammation process. However, this doesn't solve the cause of the inflammation itself. This concept is important, in order for you to achieve long term results, you need to correct as much as possible what is causing the inflammation in the first place. Even though your neck has been damaged in some way as to cause pain, it is possible to reduce the injured area thereby reducing the amount of inflammation and thus the amount of pain. As you continue to read through this book you will find many was to help you through this process. It is important for you to know what is causing your neck pain and to have consulted with your physician that reason.

Aging

It was once thought that as we age it was normal to develop stiff joints and various aches and pain resulting in a decrease in mobility. But as a normal process it does not seem to affect each individual at the same rate. This may or may not be related to injury, but perhaps a strong correlation exists. So a little common sense says that maybe this is not a natural result, or a least maybe there is something that can be done to slow the process or slow the destruction. Many proponents of anti-aging are convinced it has more to do with the overall break down of the body due to a lack of various resources, or possibly viral related as opposed to any particular aging process. There is also some thought that is may be the result of free radicals. Right now there are many areas that are being researched as to why we age the way we do. One thing that seems to have a common thread is how well we treat our bodies. There is much research that points toward the fact that our lifestyles have a great impact on how well, or how poor, we age. Which brings us to nutrition.

Alternatively speaking, pain medication has a way of depressing the immune system, and it can also cause constipation and sometimes may destroy the appetite. Anti-inflammatory drugs, as with other drugs, have side effects, adverse reactions, and drug interactions too. The long term use of these drugs can have a negative impact on your health. I think it is safe for all of us to agree that our health is important. When we are in pain, the only thing in the forefront is getting rid of that pain. However, we sometimes put our health on the back burner so that we do what we need to – get rid of the pain!

Besides eating right... you may want to consider using supplementation, herbs, or homeopathy to help with your pain. While they are no substitute for correcting the problem, they can be used as an aide. Most alternatives do not offer the side effects that prescription drugs do. As you go through this plan your overall pain should be minimized as it has been successful for many of my patients. But I want to be realistic with you; your pain would not exist if there wasn't damage done. That damage can not be totally repaired. So there will most likely be times when you feel you need to take medication to help. This is perfectly acceptable, however as time goes by, and you are faithful to the program, the need for medication will reduce. There will be things that you can do besides taking something for pain that will ultimately get you out of pain. That being said, I know it is difficult with such an array of supplements out there to know which ones are better than others. So this section of the book will help to clarify some of that information.

Supplementation is just that, you supplementing your food intake. So when someone asks you what supplements you are taking, they are most likely referring to vitamins and minerals. Homeopathy is a very dilute product that assists your body to stimulate the natural healing process. There are often no drug interactions or side effects while herbs are actually drugs that sometimes have side effects and toxic dosages, plus there may be interactions with any of the drugs you may be taking.

Supplements

Orthomolecular science is the study of vitamin therapy. Many vitamins can actually help your body to reduce your pain. Pain, in and of itself, is a stress factor. Long term stress can deplete your stores of vitamins, and put you on the deficient list. Even with the healthiest of diets, it is difficult to get all the nutrients you need simply because the quality of our soils is depleted. Thus, leaving even fresh produce lacking in the vital nutrients we need. So a good overall multi vitamin is recommended. It is also known that there are some vitamins or supplements that can help with the inflammatory process as well. These we want to take a look at.

D or DL – Phenylalanine is the _right_ handed form of a common amino acid. It is not actually a nutrient, but an amino acid analgesic in the D or DL form. Practitioners employ it for chronic pain that has been unresponsive with other measures. The dosage varies from person to person, but a good starting point is 1000 mg daily for two weeks, and increasing there after up to 3,000mg per day. After a month, if it is not helping then it probably will not, and there is no need to continue to take it. It is not addictive nor is it toxic, but as with all things do not take it if you are pregnant, consult your obstetrician. Persons with high blood pressure should take it after a meal. Persons with PKU should not take it. Those are about the only cautions with this supplement.

Vitamin C – Ascorbic Acid at high doses is known to reduce inflammation. It has natural antibiotic and antihistamine effects. Vitamin C is a water soluble vitamin and is non toxic. The best way to take it is to titrate to bowel tolerance. By this you start out taking 1000mg daily and increase the dose each day, when the first loose stool occurs then back off a dose. As you replenish your system, with time the dosage will probably decrease.

Bromelin – is an enzyme found in pineapples. It has an anti-inflammatory action that helps to reduce pain, and improves joint mobility. It is primarily used for acute injury, but also useful in arthritis. The recommended dose is 200mg per day

Ligaplex II – indications of this are for chronic joint ligament and muscular/skeletal conditions. It is important in assisting in the repair of muscle, chronic degenerative joint problems, and disc herniations. 3-6 tablets per day

Herbs

Herbal products have increased in popularity over the past 20 years, and many preparations are readily available in many of our local stores. A word of caution…herbs do have side effects, they can interact with prescription drugs, and can be toxic if not take properly. According to European Union definitions, herbal medicinal products are medicinal products containing (as active ingredients) exclusively plant material and/or vegetable drug preparations. Vegetable drugs are plant material used for a medicinal purpose in various forms as tinctures, powders, extracts, fatty or essential oils, expressed plant juices, etc. involving a purification process.

The difference between pharmaceutical medication and herbs is the overall adverse reactions and side effects. There are considerably less in herbs, plus they are natural substances found in nature whereas pharmaceutical medications are synthetic and complied in a laboratory. It is important when taking herbs that you follow the manufactures directions of recommended dosage. Overdosing is possible and each manufacture may put different strengths in their preparations.

Do not take if pregnant, consult your physician first!

White willow – 'nature's aspirin' contains salicin and comes from the inner bark of 2-3 year old white willow tree. Average <u>daily</u> dosage is 60-120 mg total salicin. Interactions with other drugs are minimal, much as what one would expect from aspirin.

Kava kava – a root herb, introduces a tranquil state, powerful skeletal muscle relaxant, eases pain and helps with depression. Average <u>daily</u> dosage is 60-120 mg kava pyrones. Interactions with other drugs may cause an increased effect of the other drug, such as alcohol, barbiturates and psychopharmacologica agents. Side effects/adverse reactions include slow motor skills. No driving or operating heavy machinery until you know how the drug effects you. Do not take for greater than three months without seeking medical advice.

Ginger – increases circulation of the blood and lymph, thus reducing swelling. It also supports a healthy response to stress and helps to maintain support of healthy joints. Ginger can be taken internally or used as a compress on the neck. Recommended <u>daily</u> dosage is 2-4 grams of rhizome (ginger root). No drug interactions or side effects are known. Contra indicated with gallstones.

Feverfew – blocks the production of the inflammatory chemicals thereby reducing inflammation and pain; also useful for migraine headaches. Take as directed by your health care provider.

Homeopathy

Homeopathic remedies stimulate the body's defenses in order to restore health. Most of the remedies are multi use. There are remedies that can be purchased in health food stores or on the internet. When choosing any remedy, be sure that the substances are listed on the bottle and the company producing it is a reputable one.

Traumeel – used for strains, sprains, inflammation, arthritis, pain, and tendonitis. Is a great modulator for pain. I have found in some patients they respond real well, others do not. One tablet dissolved under tongue three times per day.

Rhus Tox 30C – general pain remedy for most types of pain including arthritic and muscle pain and aches. Dosage is three pellets, three times per day.

While there are many preparations and combinations of herbs and supplementation as well as homeopathy, I have listed just a few of the more common ones. The combinations usually are prepared to enhance the effect or work as a synergistic component to each other. If you have questions about any preparation, call the manufacturer and talk with a sales representative. I also recommend whole food supplements as opposed to synthetic. These of course are more difficult to find but are more effective and safer.

Chapter 3

Posture: The First Step in Restoring Your Body

Posture has a significant bearing on pain and overall health. Some consider poor posture as a predisposing factor in causing many injuries. This may very well make sense when you consider that the joint can malalign with improper positioning just like the doors of a closet, famous for getting off track, so can a joint - especially when jarred. A joint is it strongest when in proper alignment and can withstand insults much easier. Recall from the previous chapters how a misaligned joint can cause inflammation, wear and tear and eventually pain. These things all put stress in your life, wear you down and deplete your energy stores. With all this in mind posture then becomes important.

A proper posture allows the body systems to function. Your heart and lungs, bowels, kidneys, liver, stomach, and all your organs and blood vessels need room to work and much like the intervertebral foramen you learned about in Chapter 1.   Any encroachment on their space will cause a problem. As an example, sit in a chair and lean forward, now take a deep breath then sit up like you would normally and take another deep breath. Did you feel the difference in your breathing…your lungs did not have very much room to expand when you are bent over, therefore you didn't breathe in enough oxygen. Since your body requires a certain amount of oxygen to function correctly, your breathing would most likely increase overtime to compensate making you work harder to get what you need.

It would seem that many people do not consider their posture to be of much significance other than to look their best. We have all been told when we were young to stand up straight, sit up straight, etc. But has anyone ever really told you why? I know that I assumed it was really more for looks than comfort. You just do not look good when you slouch. So what are the benefits of a good posture? Is it possible, now that you are an adult, to change your posture? Is it too late? To answer the latter question, it is not too late; any change is better than no change at all. As you read further you will begin to understand and learn how to correct your posture and the impact that it has on your pain level.

Many people when they stand up straight have a tendency to lift their heads up and put their shoulders back with arms down at their side. You will learn that there is a more proper way that will help to ease and relax your joints and muscles. As your first example in finding your correct posture, take a look at your present posture by looking into the mirror. In Figure 3.1 is an example of a normal posture, see if you can identify what your present posture looks like by looking at some of the samples of different postures in the pictures shown. Once you have identified your present posture, make yourself stand up straight and note what actions your body took as you did this. Did your primary movements involve throwing your shoulders back? Did you lock your knees? An important thing to realize is what is happening to you when you stand up straight without finding, what I call your 'center' first.

Figure 3.1

Normal Posture

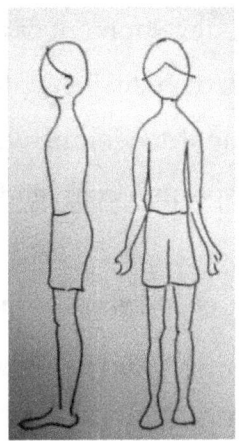

Many people when standing up straight will throw their shoulders back causing their knees to lock and more importantly increasing the natural curve of the lower back, which hyperextends and irritates the facet joints. The next thing that happens is your neck is not positioned correctly; you're either looking too far forward or downward as a counter movement to balance because your lower back is extended too far. This also would put extra stress on your body as well as bringing you out of center.

The first step in restoring your body is learning how to posture your body. It is not as simple really as standing up straight with your shoulders back and chest out, it's a little more complicated than that. Refer to Figure 3.2 and 3.3 note some of the more common abnormal postures. Just imagine how difficult it is for some of your spinal joints to function when in these positions.

With normal joint positioning the muscles on either side of a joint should be symmetric; the same on one side as the other, so if there is a misalignment, and one side is pulled too tight, the other side is not pulled enough. As you have all ready learned, this can cause irritation, muscle spasms, development of trigger points, and so on. Chronic pain may and can develop just with this factor alone. In this case the muscles are not functioning well, inflammation develops from irritation, spasms occur, and a chain reaction is initiated.

In normal posture, changes and adjustments of position are made quick and automatic. When you have poor posture you can also have problems with your organs. See Figure 3.2 for an example with a posture of kyphosis. The heart and lungs have both lost the room they were made to function in, so they can be compromised with not enough room to expand. This can cause shortness of breath or irregular heart beats, at any rate your body would have to work harder to compensate for the cramped space. It is just common sense that the harder your body is working the sooner it will wear out. Your organs that are working in a cramped space have to work harder, this means less energy for you and more fatigue.

As you can see from the Figure 3.2, the kyphotic posture also has what is termed anterior head carriage. This means the head is being carried too far forward. One recent study noted that this positioning allows hundreds of excess pounds being carried as a result from gravitational forces. That of course would add a lot of unnecessary stress to your spine.

Figure 3.2

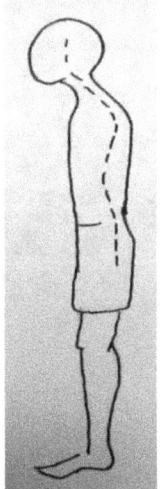

This kyphotic posture has an impact on overall health as well as adding more stress on your neck.

In summary let it be said that poor or abnormal posture can have a profound effect on your pain level, which brings us to the starting point of strengthening your neck, and because posture is a significant factor we will be working to correct your posture from feet upward. Let's address first the over standing position. On the next page are examples of some of the more common postures that we see in our everyday lives. An anatomical approach to posturing says that the stance is face forward, arms down at sides with palms of hands facing forward and feet are pointed straight out in front.

Figure 3.3

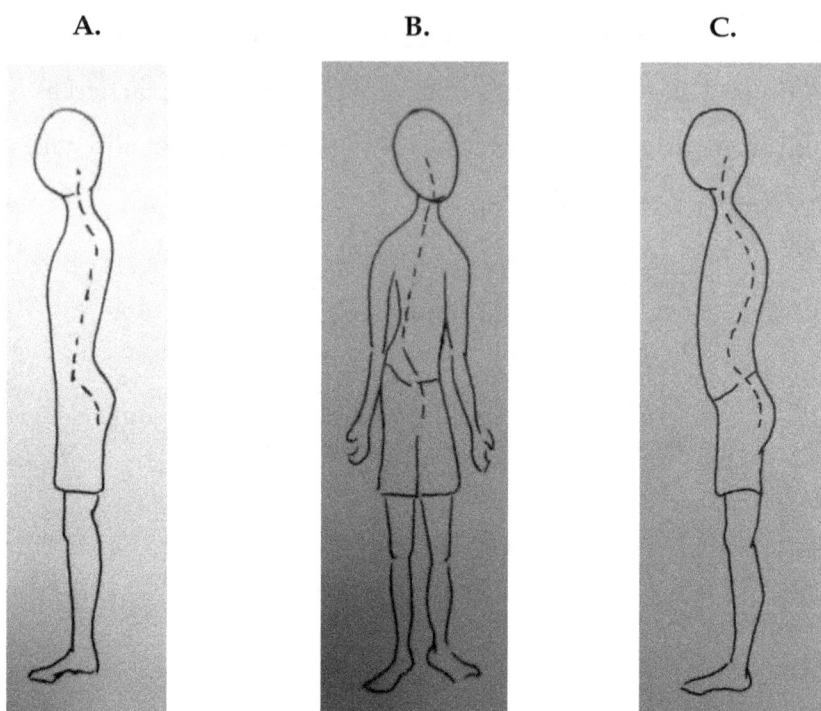

A.   **B.**   **C.**

These postures are all abnormal but common.

A. Hyperextension posture, most often seen with people who have a 'belly' but can also been seen in other people. The lower back has an excess curve often causing low back pain.

B. The common posture of Scoliosis. Note: There is an 'S' curve seen from the front instead of the side. This curve often causes over development of the muscles on the side of the stress.

C. This posture is termed "Sway Back". Usually the buttocks are flattened and the upper back is humped.

Setting up your posture

Although you may not achieve a totally normal posture, it is possible to improve upon what you do have. This will over time lessen the stresses on your body and spine. The first thing to do is to find your center. If you remember from the anatomy chapter, the natural curve of the spine, when viewed from the side, is the shape of an 'S'. When your posture is in center you avoid the excess gravitational forces upon your body unnecessarily which will promote the 'S' shape goal. You can achieve this center in two ways. The first one is the **Shoulder Shrug** and the second one is simply sitting on a **medicine ball**.

The Shoulder Shrug

The best way to do this is to stand in front of a mirror and look your self straight in the eye. This way you will not be tempted to raise or lower you head. Now gently roll both of your shoulders forward so that the backs of your hands are now at your side. Your arms are just coming along for the ride. When doing this you are **not** to move your arms – only move your shoulders forward! Your shoulders must roll to the best of their ability. Over time it will become easier and smoother. Now raise both shoulders up toward your ears, raise them as high as they will go, then gently **roll** them backwards. The palms of your hands will now be facing the front (see Figure 3.4). At this point lower your shoulders, but be careful not to let them roll forward again. With practice you will find that they will simply drop into place. I would expect that you will have to practice this several times but eventually you will be able to do this smoothly and without much thought. Take your time! If this cause pain, do it more slowly and gently. This can be repeated as often as you like, but this is not to be done so often as to cause you pain.

Figure 3.4

Exercise – Shoulder shrugs

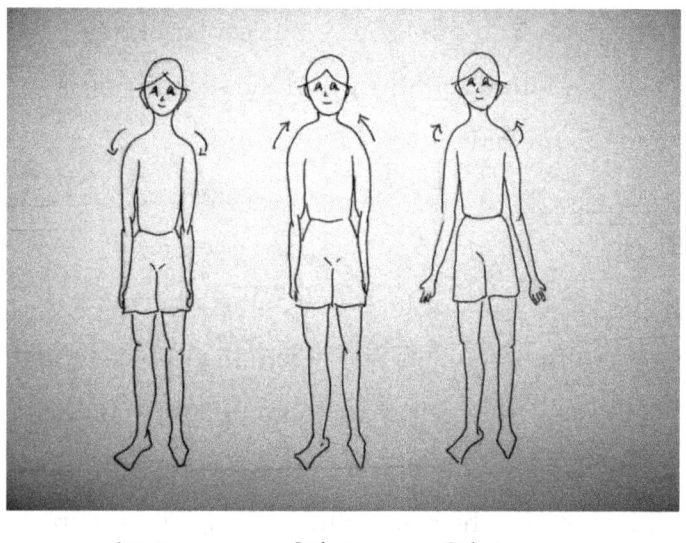

1st step   2nd step   3rd step

This exercise can be done off and on through out the day as needed. It is a good exercise not only to find your posture center, but also to relax the upper trapezium muscles. This can be done while sitting after proper technique is achieved.

Remember to roll your shoulders!

Knowing why you are doing something and getting some feedback about what you are doing will help you to keep trying, therefore some of the benefits of doing this exercise need to be explained. If posturing is done improperly, the natural curve of your lower back increases too much and can cause irritation to the facet joints. If your shoulders are not positioned right, the upper portion of the trapezium muscle begins to burn and ache, eventually impacting your neck muscles. Finding your center when standing is more proper in that it is the center for you and no one else, which means, it will help to put everything else in proportion. Slouching brings on fatigue and pain, and is often quickly identified when we read or sit in front of our computers. I blame this on the fact that a great deal of our activity is in using our arms and the projects we are working on are in front of us. Therefore, there is a tendency to roll the shoulders forward, putting us out of balance. Think of it this way, if you were to hold your arms out stretched in front of you, then you would be out of balance. And like the anterior head carriage, the force from gravity makes it very difficult for you to do this for any length of time without experiencing fatigue. If your spine is out of this 'S' shape, then parts of it are being subjected to gravity, which means that there is excess weight being carried around, again causing fatigue, stress and irritation resulting in pain. Learning how to stand up straight, in your center promotes the 'S' shape of your spine as well. Again looking at gravity, think of the 'S' shape as being a huge spring in your body that helps to absorb the shock of running, walking, and all the things we do on a daily basis. Without that 'S' shape, we are more subjected to external forces, and this can impede joint function yielding irritation and eventually pain. Your goal then is to always be in center, your center. Doing the shoulder shrugs will take you back to your center and should be repeated throughout the day. However, you must learn to do it correctly by practicing in front of a mirror while standing. The reason I ask you to do this in front of a mirror is because of your de-conditioned muscles. If you are not using a mirror it will not feel right to you and you will think you are doing it wrong. While looking into the mirror you will see that you are doing it correctly even though it does not feel right. That is the funny thing about muscles, they by now are so used to doing it the wrong way, when you do it the right way, it does not seem right. As you get more proficient at this your muscles will remember and it will then begin to feel right, then the mirror will not be needed and you will be able to accomplish the shoulder shrugs both standing and sitting.

While you are learning your shoulder shrugs you can also learn to sit on the therapy ball, or a medicine ball. These balls can be purchased at just about anywhere that sells even the smallest of exercise paraphernalia, and the cost should be somewhere around $15-$25. Most of you will need the medium - large size, if you are real tall you may want to get the next size up. Once you have purchased the ball then you need to inflate it. Do not worry, it will not bust. Inflate it as much as it will go, sometimes a measure tape comes with the ball to help determine how much to inflate. Once fully inflated, be prepared to let a little air out during sizing the ball to your height as explained in Figure 3.5.

Figure 3.5

Sizing your therapy ball

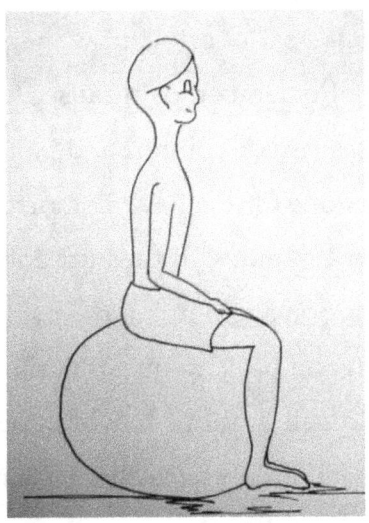

Proper height of your ball is important and it must be adjusted to fit you. You will want to be able to sit on the ball with your bare feet flat on the floor, your thighs are shooting straight out of the hips, and knees are bent at 90 degrees. See Figure 3.5. It is important that your thighs are coming out straight from your hips, neither too wide nor too narrow. The upper part of your body again needs to be in correct position, in your center. This can be accomplished by doing your shoulder shrugs then resting your hands on your lap. Your shoulders and upper arms must drop down at 90 degrees and bend at the elbow so your hands can rest in your lap. Look closely at the diagram, the shoulders are not too far forward or too far backward. Again center is important! Your head is looking straight in front - centered on your shoulders; this will occur naturally if your shoulder shrugs are done correctly. Now you are sitting in correct posture. You are now positioned on your sitting bones as you should be. Your goal is to sit this way for 20 minutes each day. A word of caution, most of you will not be able to do this at first. That's ok. Work your way up to 20 minutes. Do not sit there hurting! Remember, pain causes tissue damage, if sitting this way causes you discomfort and pain after 2-3 minutes then get up, you are done for the day. Tomorrow you will try again and see if you can do 4 minutes. If the hurt does happen, it should be relieved as soon as you stand up. If the pain is still there, then you have overdone it and back off one or two minutes the next day. However, you should still continue to work your way up again.

The rationale behind this is to strengthen your core muscles of posture. We are working with the small muscles that surround your joints - not the big ones you can see and feel. Another advantage is that this exercise will stimulate the growth of proprioreceptive fibers because of the unstable feeling of the ball. These fibers are responsible for stimulating a contraction in your muscles, acting to tighten up and hold the joint in position when you need it. A lack of these fibers can cause the contraction to be weak and therefore allow damage to the joint. After you can sit on the ball comfortably for 20 minutes, then feel free to read a book, do paper work, eat supper whatever small task you need to do while sitting on the ball, just remember to maintain your correct posture and not to get too rambunctious or you will fall off!

One more thing, the ball therapy is one of the most important things for you to do. After you have been practicing sitting on the ball for 2-3 weeks, in a very subtle way without any conscious effort on your part you will find yourself sitting in correct posture when you sit elsewhere. You may even discover that most of your living room furniture is uncomfortable to sit in. This is because your body was actually designed to sit this way. The promoting of the 'S' curve offers comfort to your tired muscles, allows your joints to be in more proper alignment and relaxed. Extra benefit - it reduces your stress!

A Final Note on Posture:

The two exercises you have just learned were designed to help you find and correct your posture as much as possible. Your body is designed to be in the 'S' shape sitting or standing. The shoulder shrug helps you to find it standing. When you sit, if you sit on your 'sitting bones', you will find this to be a 'center', it too promotes the 'S' shape and allows you to position yourself comfortably. Good posture involves training your body and muscles to stand properly, to sit properly, and even to lie down properly. The ball will help you to strengthen the muscles needed to hold you upright in proper posture - your core muscles. Although the exercises may seem simple they really work, within 2-3 weeks of daily practice you should find yourself sitting more correctly without much thought. Work with the shoulder shrugs periodically through out each day till it becomes smooth and easy. It will help you to balance, and know where to position your head and shoulders.

In Summary here are a few of the benefits of a proper posture…

➤ Reduces wear and tear allowing the body systems to function at their optimal level, there fore making you look and feel younger…this is really true. Have you ever noticed how you drag around the house when you have the flu? Take a look at how your shoulders are slumped, your feet are dragging and you are moving slowly.

➤ A centered body alignment uses the right muscles, increasing the strength of the muscle allowing for better accuracy and endurance while reducing the likelihood of injury because of an imbalance.

➤ Flexibility increases allowing joints, ligaments and muscles to operate without interference therefore maintaining the elasticity and strength. Pain begins to go away.

➤ Makes you look good!

Chapter 4

Teaching Your Body to Respond to Some New Moves (Bending, Lifting and Torque)

In the earlier chapters of this book, you learned that most problems are created by repetitive action. We are all familiar with what carpal tunnel syndrome is. This is considered an injury due to a repetitive action. Repetitive action injuries can be found in many work places where a repeated action is done for the greater part of a day...such as typing! This can be caused by the position of the body during the repetitive action. The majority of neck and back pain can be related to this type of injury. If you will remember the earlier discussion of Degenerative Disc/Joint Disease has been theorized as minor injuries that perhaps have not healed properly, but also have accumulated over time. The goal of this chapter is to teach you some new moves that will help you avoid repetitive injury, or at least reduce the amount of repetitive stresses that you put on your body by some of your everyday activity. Because there are many causes of neck pain, and many neck pains that have no causes, I should tell you that the end result is the same. All of us suffer, to some extent, from repetitive damage to our joints. If you will recall from earlier discussion that cracks and fissures within the disc can begin to occur as early as age fifteen. All of us can benefit from learning how to avoid at least some damage, which in turn, will reduce the long term effects it has on our bodies. Removing a source of irritation will in turn reduce your pain. Remember that a lot of your pain is coming from chronic irritation, and that irritation can be caused by moving incorrectly.

Sitting

As we start out, let's go back to posture. If gravity has impact on stressors that affect your body, it would stand to reason that this could be a source of repetitive damage if you are out of center frequently in the course of any given day. I refer you to the act of holding your arms stretched out in front of you. It is not very long before the arms become fatigued and start to ache and tremble. The arms are being held out from center and are subject to more gravitational force. With your arms at your side and in center you will not find it difficult or uncomfortable. When your spine gets out of the 'S' shape, that portion that is out is subjected to the same gravitational force.

If you were to sit on a couch and slouch your lower back and your neck would be out of center. Notice that most chair backs are angled slightly back (not at the required 90 degrees). This actually promotes a slouch. If you were to sit fully back into the chair and still remain on your sitting bones, the upper back would be supported and as you fatigued your lower back would slouch reversing its curve. See Figure 4.1. This in turn will allow you to extend your head backwards a little bit causing more pressure on the facets in your neck. The reason for this is that you need balance. If one part is out of place, then the other needs to balance to hold you upright. When you sit properly in the chair on your sitting bones you will discover that the back of a chair is rather useless.

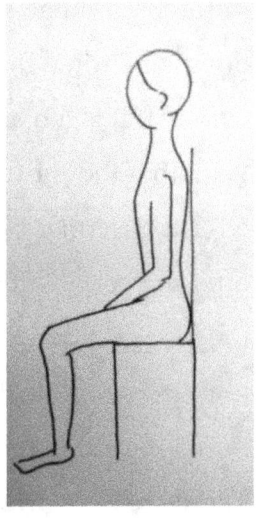

Figure 4.1

Notice that the chair has a straight back to it. The feet are flat on the floor, thighs are parallel to the floor, and arms are bent comfortably at the elbow and resting on the lap.

At first this may not seem possible but as you practice sitting on your therapy ball you will find that you instinctively assume this position when sitting elsewhere. Since gravity produces stress on your body, when you are out of your center you can see that over time an injury would result because of the weight of gravity would put an extra stressors on your ligaments and tendons. After enough of this, they may weaken or fibers may become torn and the joint becomes more susceptible. A slight change in the biomechanics of its motion will begin to happen, and over more time pain will result as the injuries become more pronounced and are not healing well. The small little injuries become big injuries and now you are stuck with chronic pain.

I have seen and heard that a solution to sitting and supporting your back might be to place a pillow in the small of your back, this will help but you must remember that the pillow needs to fit you perfectly which is difficult since we are all created a little different. When supporting your curves in this fashion either laying down or sitting, the pillow must fit perfectly in order to keep the 'S' curve. If it is too large or too small then you will alter the curve. With that thought in mind, there are supports out there that are adjustable either by water or by an air pumped apparatus. These offer the best solutions because of their adjustability of fitting you to the proper depth. Now, if you choose to use supports, then it is important to note that prolonged use of supports will decrease your muscle strength that you are replacing with the back support. There are industries out there that have their employees wear harnesses and such things to offer back supports because their jobs require lifting. However, studies have shown that this is not as effective in preventing injury as once thought. The reason for this is because constant wearing of the support allows the muscles to become weakened since they no longer are needed. Our bodies have a slogan if you will…"use it or loose it", so if the back support is doing the job of the muscles, then the muscles do not have to work and they will not. Simple - but true. The same theory would apply to anything that you do. As you begin to place a demand of your core muscles to support you in proper posture (like sitting on the ball) you are demanding core muscle support, which your body will comply with, over time. This kind of explains why your muscles are de-conditioned. The demand has been placed on the wrong muscle.

Driving

Another common sitting position that causes damage is when you drive a car. This will probably have a significant impact on you because of your neck pain. To demonstrate the effect of gravity, find a chair that suits you, having the same size as your ball in that you are able to place your feet flat on the floor and your knees are bent at 90 degrees. If the chair is too tall or too short this test will not work, so be sure to find the proper chair. Position yourself in your sitting posture just as if you were to sit on your ball. Stay like this for about one minute. Now move your arms slightly forward on your lap. It doesn't have to be very far, just enough to get you out of center. As you do this, pay attention to the shift in weight. You should notice that as you move your arms forward in your lap that the weight shifts to your upper back across your shoulders. You are out of center now and gravity has got a hold of you. Another test that will demonstrate this is to assume the correct sitting position again only this time lean back into the chair so your upper back is resting against the chair. This time the weight shifted to your lower back.

Now when you drive a car your hands have to hold the steering wheel and more often than not the position of the seat is too far away causing your hands and arms to be way out of center. This is the reason that the back of your neck and shoulders begin to ache and burn after any time of driving. So to minimize the damage, try to position the seat in your car as close to proper positioning as possible. When you do take long trips, you should take frequent breaks from driving because of this factor. I make it a point to stop at every rest stop available, just to get out walk around for a minute, get back in the car and be on the road again. I have found that this helps a great deal. Another useful trick is to make use of the arm rest and the console of the car by alternating resting positions frequently, and to use both arms and hands to steer. I also do my shoulder shrugs to keep the upper trapezium from tightening up too much. As a general rule, try to stop and get out of the car at least every hour or so. Going much over that you will probably begin to feel achy which will usually result in that burning feeling in your neck and shoulders. That burning may become a full blown flare up of your pain.

By now you should be getting a good picture that one of your stressors that increase your pain has been the position you are using while sitting. It would seem that it may be impractical to at all times be in proper sitting posture, but your goal is to reduce the number of incorrectness. When you are fatigued at the end of the day, by all means use pillow supports to help. One of the best pieces of living room furniture to invest in is a winged back chair. They are built with their backs at 90 degrees. When you add a footstool, you will find that it is a pretty comfortable position. If you are slouching a little then put a small pillow in the lower back, one that has the proper depth to fill in the hollow of your lower back. The winged back chair offers support for your head because it is high enough, and will take the pressure of off your neck. It makes a much better option than most couches or easy chairs.

Standing

The next position to look at is standing. Obtaining a more correct standing posture helps to get you into position for bending as well as endurance when standing in line or other such things. If you will notice that many people stand with their legs parallel or straddle to one another as in Figure 4.2. It is not that this position is necessarily a bad position, but that there is a better one. The stance I like is what is called a scissor stance. See Figure 4.3. This stance will be of benefit when circumstances warrant that you have to stand for any length of time, or there is a need to bend. This will increase your center, allowing for greater stability. This also gives you strength that you can elicit from your torso more readily.

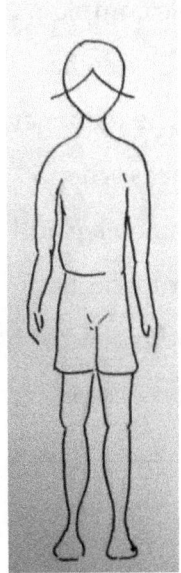

Figure 4.2

This stance is very common and is used when doing your shoulder shrugs, however for standing positions of any length the scissor stance should be used.

As an example try each position your self and notice how the scissor stance is more comfortable and more stable. When bearing your weight on either leg, you also notice that the stress on your hips has lessened. Since you cannot lock your knees, the stress on your lower back is gone. Now while in the scissor stance try a shoulder shrug putting you totally in center.

Figure 4.3

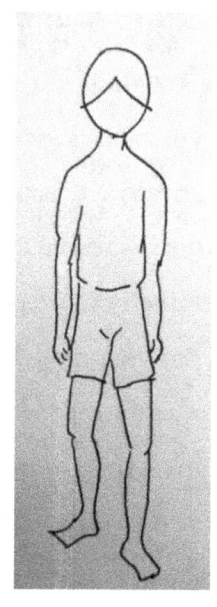

Notice that the feet are no longer parallel when standing. One foot is comfortably placed behind the other. This stance widens the platform, and allows for better balance, which reduces stress on your hips and knees.

I am sure that you have often heard many people complain of back aches after standing for long periods. Again, look at what happens if you are using the parallel/straddle stance. The tendency is to lock the knees. It is a little difficult to soften the knees when standing this way. You will either put all the weight on one leg and stress the hip, or you will lock the knees and cause your lower back to hyperextend. Now when the lower back hyperextends (bends backwards too much) the rest of your body will want to balance, that means your neck is going to get out of center too! As another example take a look at someone who is pregnant. The weight of the belly causes the woman to hyperextend her lower back to balance herself (frequent backaches because her facets are too close together causing irritation). Then take a look at the position of her head and note that it will be slightly bent forward causing her neck to be out of center as well. In a pregnant woman this will be a temporary position, once the baby is born there will be no need for her to adapt her stance, and she will without thought revert back to her previous posture be it good or bad.

Figure 4.4

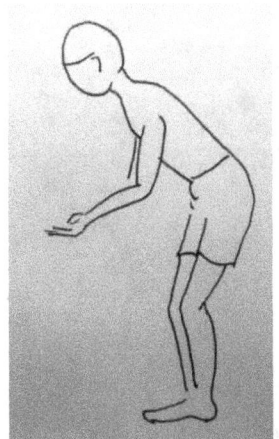

Most of us learned to bend with our knees bent, keeping our back straight. However, this seems to be more difficult. When simply bending to retrieve objects from a height such as a table, most will round their backs even with the knees bent! Compare this with Figure 4.5

With the scissor stance you are primed for bending. Bending should be done at the hip joint - not at the back. If you bend down to retrieve your car keys off of the kitchen table, and you are not in the scissor stance, your lower back will reverse its curve. If on the other hand you are in the scissor stance, the tendency will be to pivot at your hip instead of your back ,and at the same time your knees will bend. To exemplify this more, set your keys on the seat of a chair as this is lower than a table and will be more pronounced. Try bending to pick up your keys in both positions and note the difference. Once you have done this and can readily identify the difference in your lower back, do it again and note the different position your neck automatically reverts too. You should see that your neck maintains a proper position when you use the scissor stance as well.

Figure 4.5

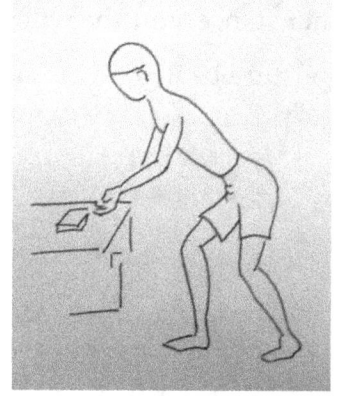

Notice that when using the scissor stance to bend, the lower back is kept more straight and the knees are bent. You will also find that your neck does not flex as much either. This particular stance is more appropriate when bending or lifting.

Again this is very subtle, but with time can be a source of irritant because of the number of times you bend throughout the day. It isn't about heavy lifting at all. It could be something as simple as picking up a small object from a surface that is lower, thus causing you to bend ever so slightly could be cause of pain. If you think about it, most of us when preparing to lift, do just that we psyche ourselves and position our bodies hopefully in the right manner. But when lifting a piece of paper off of a table, we just do not think of that as lifting. Bending, such a simple act, but if done incorrectly can result in repetitive damage and irritation. Practice this new move with lots of examples you can think of that you do routinely, and note how you are doing it. Then correct it by using the scissor stance and watch for the difference. I think you will be pleasantly surprised.

Neck pain sufferers, just like low back sufferers, can find lifting painful too. If you watch anyone lifting a heavy object, look at how they can use their necks for leverage. They are not really using the neck as much as the weight of the head. We have often heard someone say bend your knees when you pick up something, which something is usually referring to an object that is heavy. The truth of the matter is that with the straddle position and our knees bent we often round our lower backs and hunch our shoulders forward when getting in position to pick up something heavy. It takes effort for us to keep our backs straight and head looking forward. However, when using the scissor stance you will find that you have greater strength and more balance when lifting. The scissor stance should be wider than when just bending over to retrieve something off a table or chair. See Figure 4.6

Figure 4.6

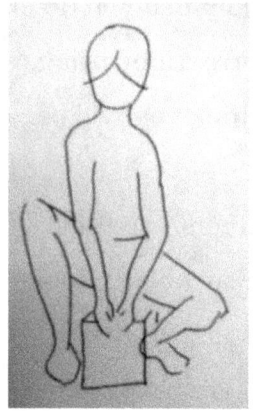

Notice how close to the object you can get when picking up. Because you are close to the object it becomes part of your center, you also have more leverage and balance causing less stress and energy.

Figure 4.7

Using your knee to place the object can be of benefit if the object is heavy. When done properly it will allow you leverage of your torso as opposed to just using your back. Also note how your neck can stay in alignment, but also because your head is so much in the widened center the pressure will not be as great on your neck.

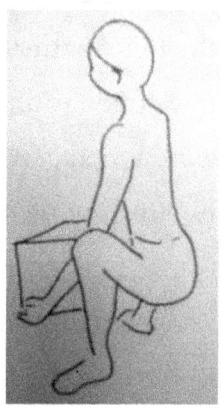

Practice first bending in the usual position with straddled stance, as if you were going to pick up a box off the floor, then practice using the scissor stance. You will have to make sure the scissor is wide enough; your stance could almost engulf the box so that perhaps a portion of it fits between your legs. Now as you move your arms forward, as if to pick up the box, note that your shoulders cannot round as much because they fit between your legs.

Thus, you will have to pivot on your hips as you lean forward with arms ready to pick up the box. This keeps both your neck and lower back in a more correct position. Also the stance is more balanced and there is not too much danger of you loosing your balance when you realize it is heavier than what you thought! If you are picking up a small box that is rather heavy, you can use your thigh as a sort of table, then use the momentum of your torso to pick yourself up to standing. Using your torso when lifting will give you greater strength than using your back or neck. That is the whole point. Try practicing with small objects first then graduate to heavier things.

Another way to use your torso is when you have to push or pull something. Again with the scissor stance, widened as when lifting from the ground, hunker down to the level of what you are going to push or pull then rock back on your foot. Use the front foot if you are pulling, the back foot if you are pushing. This will enable you to put your body weight behind the effort and lessen the effect on your neck and shoulders.

Torque

One of the things that cause the most stress on your spine is what is termed a shearing force. In terms of gravitational weight the most stress that is put on your spine occurs when you are sitting. Standing is in the middle, while lying down is the least. When our bodies are in neutral (face forward, torso forward and feet pointed forward) that is one particular weight, but as soon as we twist it then it produces a shearing force upon the spine. This combined with the weight of gravity, becomes a stressor and over time a repetitive injury.

Consider sitting at a desk, facing forward and the telephone is to the right. Each time you pick up the telephone your body twists to reach the phone and bring it to your ear. This is a shearing force upon the spine. Let us consider another example. You are at the kitchen sink filling a pan of water, facing the sink directly with feet straddle. Once the pan of water is full you are going to place it on the counter. As you do this your torso twists to put the pan on the counter beside the sink. Ouch!

Figure 4.8

This parallel stance is too rigid to allow a complete turn of your body therefore the waist will twist to finish the move creating a shearing force.

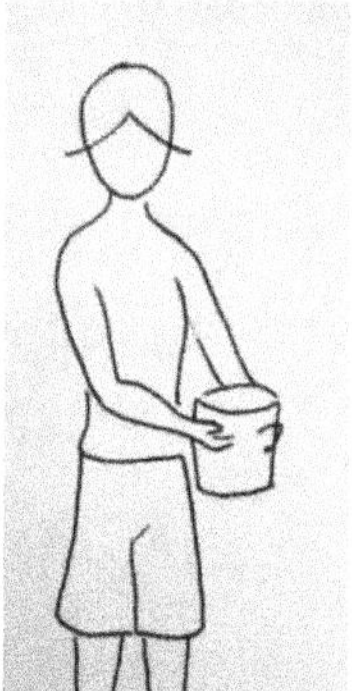

Again a shearing force has been created and with the pan of water, you have also loaded the spine with more weight. So with the feet parallel to one another and twisting the body without moving our feet we create a term called torsion or torque. Over time, as with any repetitive motion, creates a trauma or injury. When the scissor stance is utilized in place of the parallel stance your feet will automatically pivot as you begin to turn your torso, and will avoid the loaded shearing force.

Figure 4.9

When comparing with figure 4.8 you can see the torso is more turned to the activity at hand.

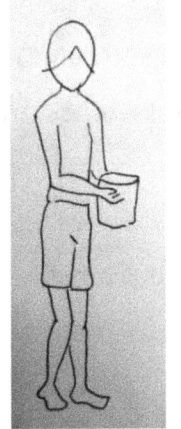

You are at the sink filling the pan with water. Your feet are now scissored with the right foot behind. As you lift the pan to put it on the counter, your right foot will pivot as your torso turns to the right to place the pan of water on the counter. Now it can be said that with the parallel position of your feet that when placing the pan of water to the right of you that your left foot will pick up a little allowing your body to turn with the pan of water. However, considering that your center is widened with the scissor stance you will actually have more strength to lift the pan of water, therefore the weight response is lessened as well as the ability for more distance before torque occurs. Test this out with a few things around the house, and you will see that this is a much better stance that reduces the over all load on your spine and therefore the overall stress and injury.

Summary

Some of the most common things that we do through out the day cause many of our stresses to the spine and neck, the way we hold our head, the way we bend, twist, and perform many of the activities of daily living. The concept is to minimize the overall damage by altering the way we do things. So far we have addressed posture and its effects. Maintaining correct posture as we do things is important not just when we are standing or sitting, but also when we bend or twist. This sounds like an insurmountable task, but it really is quite simple and becomes common place after just a few weeks of practice.

By knowing the concept and theory you can begin to evaluate a situation, and then put into practice what you have learned. Thus far we have discussed standing, sitting, and twisting. As in so many things, most of what is common place creates problems. Let us consider the standard chair. As all ready noted most chairs have their backs slanted at a small degree meaning that they do not form a 90 degree angle. The angle of the chair then is not conducive to helping you sit up straight. This is why you get off of your sitting bones using the back of the chair for support. If done properly the back of the chair will not be needed, but if you are sitting in the chair far enough back and are on your sitting bones you will find that your upper back is somewhat supported by the back of your chair and this is ok as long as you maintain sitting on your sitting bones. The problems is when you begin to get fatigued you will slouch and reverse the curve in your lower back and to a certain degree cause your neck to 'hyperextend', pressing in on those facet joints. So as the length of time is increased a pillow support maybe helpful to avoid getting out of center, but use this only for periods of relaxation choosing a chair that can also support your head, then adjusting yourself to center as much as possible. During working hours it is best to rely on posture muscles, as this will continue to strengthen and tone your core muscles. Do not forget to use your shoulder shrugs periodically and take frequent breaks to alter static positioning as you work. These efforts will help to decrease the amount of stresses placed on your neck, thereby decreasing irritation and finally your pain.

Chapter 5

The Workplace

Some reports indicate that nearly 23,000 work-related neck injuries caused employees to miss work. This can be a little tricky because you do not want to lose your job, be thought ill of because you miss work due to pain, or cannot accomplish your work because of your pain. I think that most of us by now are familiar with hazards of not obtaining employment because of a history of back injury. The same holds true with neck injuries. But with chronic neck pain it is not necessary to lift anything for us to hurt; we just have to sit there.

Since there seems to be an abundance of desk workers we will start there. The principles are the same really no matter what the job, so if you do not work at a desk read this chapter any way. The key to preventing the pain from reoccurring is to properly design your work space. This really pertains to any type of work. The goal is to have your work station fit you and adapt to you. Not the other way around. I realize that this may not be possible for a lot of people, but given the principles and a little ingenuity you may be able to come close, or at least closer, than your present situation. As you read through, I suggest you compare each of the recommended positions, or methods, with your current work place. This way you can make sure that you are on the right path.

Let's begin with your chair. If you will remember your therapy ball, this is the same position you need for your chair. As a review your feet must be flat on the floor, legs shoot straight out of the hips, and are parallel to the floor; knees are bent at 90 degrees. This will help you determine what the height your chair needs to be. Most chairs these days are height adjustable. The problem comes when you are too short, or too tall, and the desk doesn't match. If you find that you are too short in this position for your desk, then readjust the chair to match the desk and use a foot rest. There are available commercial ones that can be adjusted for height or you can make your own. Words of caution...some of the commercial foot rests I have seen allow you to rest your feet in a vertical or semi vertical position, not flat on the floor. If it does not fit flat on the floor then choose another because this will cause your lower back to reverse its curve, therefore causing a lack of support for the lower back, which may cause you to develop lower back problems. This is definitely not the goal; you are trying to keep within your center and maintain as much of your 'S' curvature as possible.

Once you have your chair at the proper height, now notice your elbows. Your arms should hang straight down from the shoulder at 90 degrees and bend at the elbow - 90 degrees in front of you. This would be the proper height of your desk, at minimum where your keyboard lies. If your chair has arms, and they can be positioned, it would be appropriate to adjust the chair arms to rest your arms on. This way you will not find yourself leaning over to rest your arm on the arm of the chair. The height of the desk can be a real problem. You may have to place your desk on blocks at each of the legs to accommodate the proper height, or a platform can be built to allow your feet to rest on. As mentioned earlier, the height needs to be the same as the height when you sit and bend your elbows 90 degrees. This allows your body to stay in proper position. Sitting on your sitting bones this will help to promote your center. By now having practiced sitting on the ball you should not have any difficulty finding the correct position when sitting.

Figure 5.1

In this diagram please note that due to the simplicity the feet do not appear flat on the floor and the thighs do not appear to be parallel to the floor. This should be one of your considerations when choosing your chair. Feet flat, thighs parallel. Also, note how close the table is and at what level it is in relation to the torso. This is better, because you are putting less strain on your neck and shoulders.

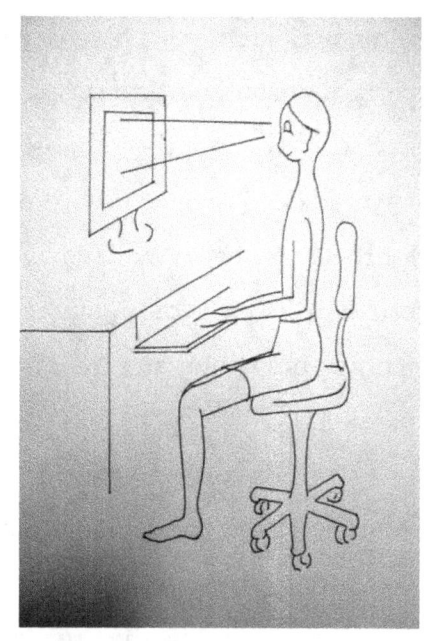

As you can see from the above diagram this position simulates your same position on the ball. Ball sitting is the first thing you must be able to do, usually in about two weeks, you will be able to sit comfortably on the ball in the correct position. If you find that sitting in proper position at work is uncomfortable then use the same strategy as when you started the ball. Probably the most difficult positioning will be your head, but as you are practicing your shoulder shrugs and getting better at it, you will find that your head will naturally position itself in the correct form, but again this takes practice.

The best form of desk is an L-shaped desk and a swivel chair on wheels. I say this because having to turn your head frequently can often cause more pain. The best example I can think of is for those of you that do copy work, by this I mean you are inputting information into a computer and having to look over at the information while you type into the computer. There are arms that will attaché to the computer that will hold your copy directly in front of you. If at all possible you want to be able to keep you head in a neutral position, facing forward. See Figure 5.1. The swivel chair will allow you to pivot in the chair and not use your neck to do this. The phone is also another matter. With a swivel chair you will be able to once again pivot the chair, face forward to answer the phone, all without torque to your neck or torso.

Another advantage of an L-shaped desk is that it gives you another work station. Your computer is set up on one side of the L, and a cleared space is available on the other side. This allows you to be able to sit squarely in front of any project you have to do that does not involve your computer, or that you may be doing both, inputting at different points etc. With a chair that can pivot, you will not torque as much, therefore the shearing effect that occurs with this action is avoided causing less irritation to the spine and neck. If an L-shaped desk is not an option, try creating your workstations close together so you can pivot from one function to the other. Keep in mind that your goal is not to torque, or twist, your neck when you alter your position to handle different tasks. With these concepts in mind you should be able to adjust your present workstation to accommodate.

Just to reiterate, we have discussed desk height, chair position, and the desktop. Now lets us go into what height your computer screen should be. When you first started practicing your shoulder shrugs, you needed to look in the mirror to keep the position of your head correct as you watched to make sure you were doing it right. The same concept holds true here, when facing a mirror and looking at yourself straight in the eyes your head is in neutral. Neither too far bent forward or backward. The same should hold true of your computer screen. One of the worst positions for your neck is to have your head bent backwards causing excess pressure on your facets which will soon become irritated. Bending forward puts stress on your lower neck and shoulders. Both of these irritants will by the end of the day create more pain.

It will be bit easier to adjust the height of the computer if you do not have a lap top. The desk top computer screens all have a base which is some what adjustable to be able to tilt backwards or forwards, and if need be, to put a book under it to raise the overall height. If you were to simulate the position at home just to get the feel it would look like something in Figure 5.2.

Figure 5.2

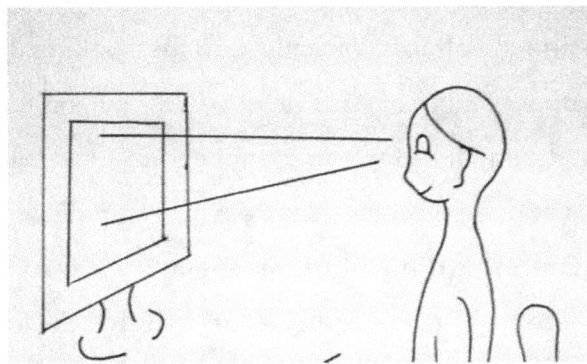

This is what is termed eye level. When in this position it is not necessary to bend your neck up or down. A movement of your eyes will be enough.

The laptop computer is much more difficult to adjust, but is becoming more and more common because of its portability. The more important aspect of adjustment for this type of computer would be your elbow and forearm position. Resting the computer on top of the desk will most certainly raise you arms upward to type and force you to bend your head forward to view the screen. Often time's desks will come with a pull out shelf that is designed to hold the keyboard and this seems to be a pretty appropriate height for arm placement as well, while the monitor is placed on the desktop. If your desk has a pull out shelf consider placing the laptop there for a short period, then move it to the desk top, sort of back and forth to alter the position you are working in therefore reducing the stress of long term incorrect positioning. In either case you will want to be sitting as close to the computer as possible to avoid the neck shoulder stress that will come to pass as the day goes on. By sitting closely you may be able to point your elbows outward resting them on the desktop while you type. Your head can be positioned almost correctly, and just looking down without a downward movement of your head will allow you to see the screen. The temptation will be for you to move your head into a downward position as you are working. Those who wear glasses or bifocals, you will have more difficulty adjusting to the screen at this level. The awkwardness here of course is the fact that the keyboard and screen are inseparable.

Another solution to the laptop dilemma might be the use of two computers if you have that option. Let us say that you bring a lot of work home, thus the portability of the laptop. If possible you could transfer data at the end of the day to the laptop thereby making your primary computer the desktop model; this would reduce your overall stress factors that ensue with the laptop, which brings us to another problem…briefcases, book bags, etc. Since the portability of the laptop, a lot of commuters are carrying quite a load to and fro. Some of them do it all on one shoulder. This is not a good thing. Ever tried to pick up a child's book bag?

Wheels can be the solution. Although I am told by most students that this is not very 'cool', but it certainly is much more practicable. With the wheels, you only have to lift it in and out of the car. The rest of the time it can be rolled and you avoid the stress of the extra weight which is often awkward to carry in the first place. We talk a lot about balance, so if something such as a book bag or brief case has to be carried it will need to be balanced. This is not an easy task. Luggage and such things are often bulky and no two bags weigh the same. The use of wheels will allow you to be more versatile even though there will be times when you cannot use them. So if you are to carry 10 pounds in one hand, then ten pounds need to be carried in the other hand for balance. If you are to carry a book bag, then carry it on both shoulders to even out the weight. See Figure 5.3.

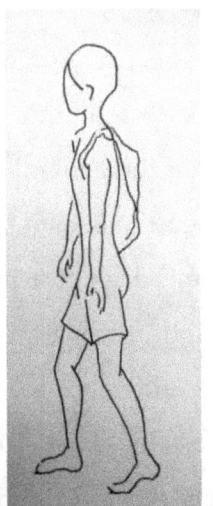

Figure 5.3

Note the book bag is carried on both shoulders.

Have you ever noticed that hikers carry all their gear on both shoulders? They also have a strap from their back packs that goes around their waist; this distributes the weight even more and puts less weight directly on the shoulders and spine. Since most book bags do not have a waist option getting one with wheels would help. If the bag you carry is more of the brief case style then use the shoulder strap that comes with it to carry the bag, the shoulder strap is crossed over your chest onto the opposite shoulder, this distributes the weight more onto your torso then directly on one shoulder. See Figure 5.4.

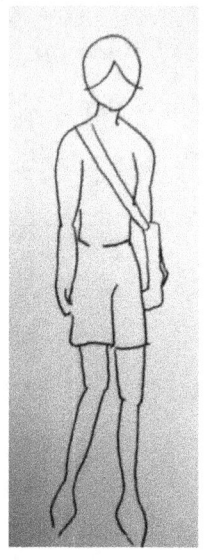

Figure 5.4

The strap on the shoulder bag is crossed over the opposite shoulder.

The designers of luggage, carry-on bags, book bags, etc. can sometimes design things that are ergonomically sound, but if the general public will not use it the way it was designed, then the design often gets lost in the shuffle. I see all the time that people are not using things the way they were meant to. It is a rare sight to see a man in a three-piece suit carrying a book bag on both shoulders, or for that matter, carrying his brief case with the strap across his chest. More often than not, he has a carry-on that he is wheeling behind him, he is carrying his laptop on the opposite shoulder, or hand, and his spine is bent towards the side that has the most weight. The neck and head then would be bent towards the side that with the least amount of weight…to balance. Would it not have been better to carry the laptop in a more ergonomically sound way or even to tie it in some manner to the luggage that has wheels? A little ingenuity goes a long way; your goal is, as always, to reduce the amount of stress to your neck, back and shoulders. If you reduce the amount of irritation, then you will reduce the amount of pain you have on a daily basis. You are learning great concepts, and these concepts can be applied to most anything you encounter. Take the time to think about it. Soon it will be an integral part of you, and you will just do it.

Another issue is that of repetitiveness and static. When we are really involved in something, we can go at it for 2-3 hours before we break. This is not a good thing! It is important to switch positions frequently. This frequency is about two times each hour. As an example, suppose you are typing away, the project is flowing nicely and your mind is 100 percent on target. About 20 minutes into the project, stop a minute, do a shoulder shrug, stretch your neck, maybe stand up and walk around your chair, then sit and resume your position and go at it again. By doing this you have disrupted your stasis and have stimulated blood flow and allowed tissues to stretch and alter their position. This is actually a healthy thing to do, and will allow you to work for a longer period of time without irritation. The point is to break the static. Get up go to the copier; go get a drink of water, just something to break the static.

Most of our discussion in this chapter has been on office type workers, while I realize that there are many other types of workers, the concepts remain the same. Your goal is to keep yourself in center, and to minimize the amount of stress to your neck. This can be accomplished even if your job requires you to lift, drive, stand, walk, etc...doesn't matter the concepts and principles are the same. The repetitive action over time will cause irritation, and that irritation results in tissue damage and scar tissue. This will happen time after time, till the joint can no longer function correctly because of the damage. Minimize the irritation, and then minimize the damage and the pain. It may be that you feel there is nothing that can be done about your workplace because you have no say. This is not totally true, most employers need you to work and within reason can accommodate minor changes to your workstation.

Now, let us go over some of the concepts that you have learned and try to imagine how you can adapt each concept to your lifestyle, at work and at home.

1.   Stance – positioning yourself when standing upright, use the scissor stance for more balance and distribution of weight

2.   Sitting – centered on your sitting bones, thighs shooting straight out the hip, knees bent 90 degrees with feet flat on the floor, shoulders and head are centered, elbows are bent at your waist and forearms resting comfortably on your lap

3. Bending – using scissor stance pivoting at the hip joint keeping the 'S' curve of your spine, facing whatever you are to pick up directly, not angled.

4. Lifting – wide scissor stance, bending down to the floor using thigh and hip, not back, arms are positioned between legs to keep shoulders and neck from straining.

5. Twisting – torque and torsion, use the scissor stance to ensure back foot pivots with motion and allows the torso to evenly turn in the direction of motion

These are your primary moves, and are to be done daily, if not more frequently. These moves will eventually become an integral part of what you do - you will not even think about it.

Chapter 6
Strengthening and Exercise

A study in the Journal of American Medical Association revealed that a regular exercise program of strengthening the muscles of the neck reduced pain, increased mobility, and required less analgesic medication. Although there are many causes of neck pain, some of which we have previously discussed, many people with chronic neck pain have no known cause. It has been said, and as research continues, stress alone can often be a predisposing factor in the development of chronic neck pain. This chapter begins your stretching and strengthening. These exercises are designed to be incorporated into your daily activities. This is important, you must do these daily. We have specified that a lot of the exercises can be done throughout the day, especially if you are in pain. At no point should pain be created. If an exercise causes you pain, then do it again in front of the mirror to be sure your technique is correct. If pain continues, then stop the exercise and try again at another time. Because your muscles are weakened, and out of shape, you should begin these exercises slowly and within your tolerance level. At first you may only be able to handle slight movements, but with practice, as the muscles improve, your movements will become stronger and better.

Range of Motion

This should be accomplished prior to moving forward!

To begin, you first should be able to do range of motion which is the ability to be able to bend your head forward, backwards, bend side to side, and turn side to side. When you begin with movement of your head and neck in its range, you may find that it does not move well - this is ok. What you want to do is to move in the range that is tolerable up to the start of pain. Then inch into the pain just slightly, and stop. That is it. You can do more tomorrow! By the end of a week you should be able to go through your range, and show an increase in that range that is not painful. Try to measure your progress it is helpful.

Stretches

Stretches help to relieve pain and discomfort, but only if done right. They must be soft and easy. Stretch to a point that you just begin to feel a slight burn, then stop and hold. Count to 15 then stretch just a tiny bit more and count again to 15. Then go on to the next muscle.

CAUTION: Do not push with your stretches. Neck muscles are fragile and over stretching will cause a spasm. So go gently forward!

Scalenus stretches

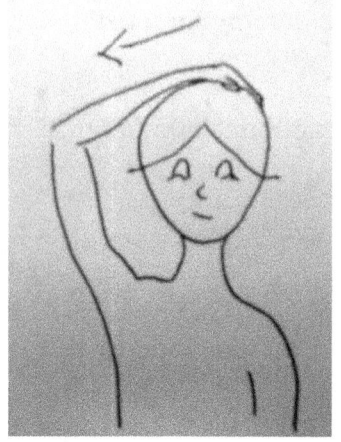

Looking straight ahead, take the pads of your fingers and gently pull your head towards your upheld arm.

Turning your head toward your upheld arm, take the pads of your fingers and pull towards your same upheld arm.

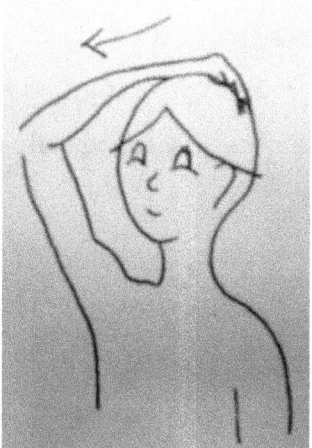

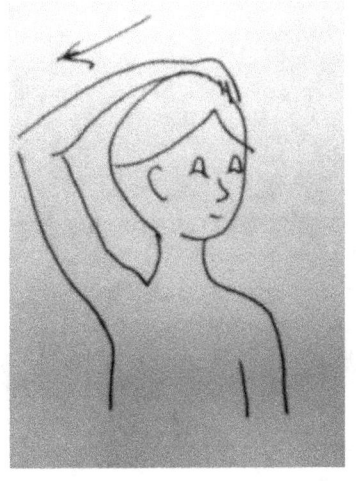

Now turn your head in the opposite direction, away from your upheld arm. Pulling with the pads of your fingers, pull your head towards the upheld arm.

That is a total of 3 stretches on each side, be gentle and do not force the movement, as your muscles improve so will the stretch. After doing one side then take your other arm and repeat for the other side. The stretches are only to be held in place for a count 20-30, and then gently return your head back to neutral. If your neck hurts then you have gone too far. Some will only be able to stretch a little bit at first. That is ok! It will improve with practice. With each turn of the head, and stretch, you should feel each at a different location. Remember there are three muscles here that you are stretching. If your range of motion is not normal, such as not turning your head as far right as you can left, then do it within the range that you have. With time and patience your range may eventually increase.

Frog Stretch

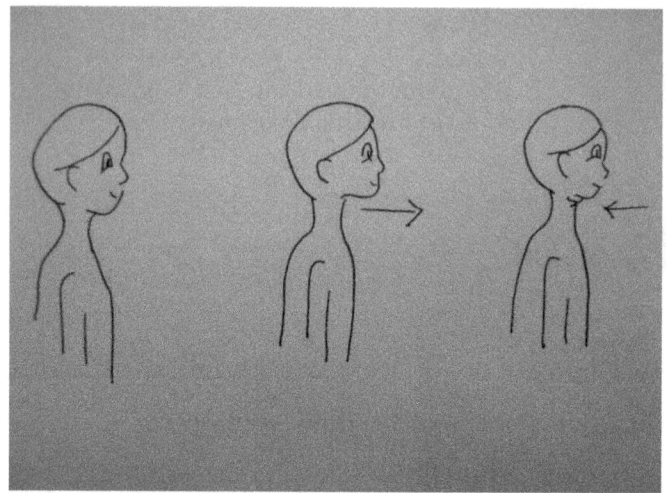

This stretch is for the two back muscles from the spinalis group. At the end move, your chin should double.

While holding your head in neutral, stretch forward keeping your head level and in the neutral position. It is real easy to lift your head up or down so be careful to keep it level or in neutral position. Stretch as far as you can go, then bring you head (keeping it straight) back as far as it will go, then hold for 20-30 seconds and your done. When in the back position, your chin should be doubled, this way you will know you have gone back far enough. The stretch should be felt in the back of the neck along either side of your spine and against the base of your skull. This is a nice stretch to do while driving or at work.

So far we have done simple range of motion and stretches. The stretches have covered the major muscles in the neck that will cause problems. Once you have accomplished these stretches then do a couple of shoulder shrugs to relieve the tension in the upper trapezium and you are done. These should, and can be done, throughout the day. When your neck begins to hurt, these exercises will often relieve the pain. But be careful, over doing will create pain, so move forward slowly.

Just for review I have included the shoulder shrug:

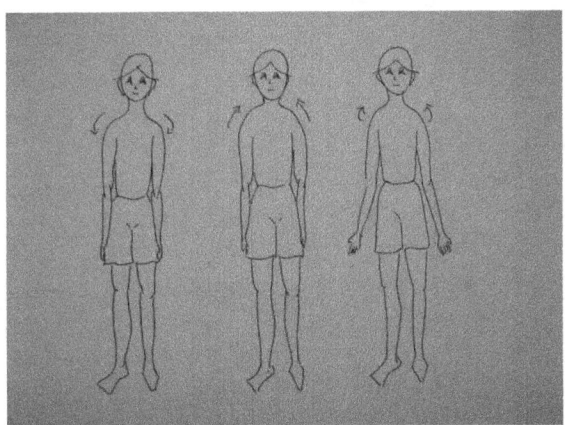

Standing in a parallel stance, roll shoulders forward. While your shoulders are rolled forward, raise the shoulders toward your ears as high as they will go. Now, roll the shoulders backward, then down till you feel a 'clunk'. This is your center. Be careful not to let your shoulders return to the old position. As a side note you can do 2-3 quickly and in a succession, this will relax the upper muscles across the top of your shoulders causing goose bumps and relaxing the muscles. The shoulder shrug also helps you to find out how to hold your head and will actually stop the pain when placed in center.

The next exercises, after you are proficient and can do the previous exercises without pain, are termed resistive exercises. Applying tension to your head and attempting to move against the strength of your hand will allow for a gentle resistance of the movement and strengthen your neck muscles. Again, caution is needed and although it doesn't seem like a lot, remember these muscles are fragile and will easily strengthen with resistive exercises. It will also increase tone of the muscle. Your goal is to strengthen and tone the muscles allowing for smoother operation of movement, in turn reducing irritation and pain. These exercises are not designed to create bulk in the muscle.

Note: Starting position is always with head in neutral position.

Resistive exercises

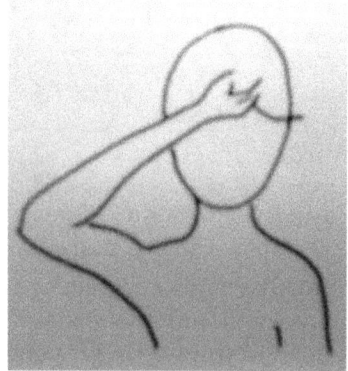

Extension (bending head backward)
Place your hand on the back of your head and push your head into your hand. Your hand should be around the crown of your head. Push the head into your hand, and then relax. Repeat this process 2-4 times. As an alternative you can do this particular one against a wall by standing in center with your back as close to the wall as possible and instead of pushing into your hand, push into the wall.

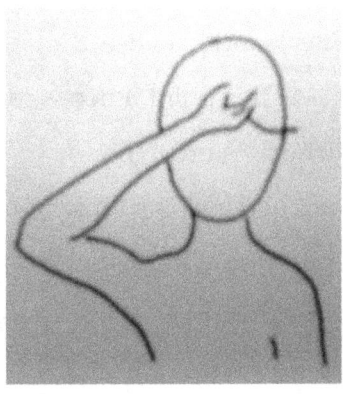

Flexion (bending head forward)

With your head in neutral, place your hand on your forehead. Now push your head forward into your hand. Then relax your head after 2-3 seconds. Repeat 2-4 times to tolerance.

Lateral flexion (bending head sideways)

With head in neutral place, place hand on one side of the head. Now push head into hand for 2-3 seconds then relax. Repeat 2-4 times to tolerance. Do same procedure on the other side.

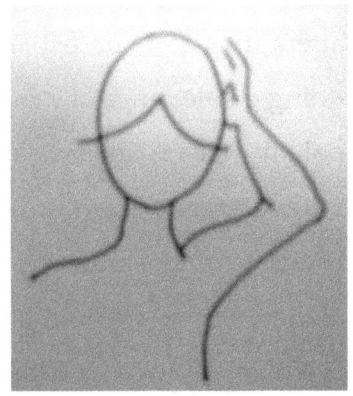

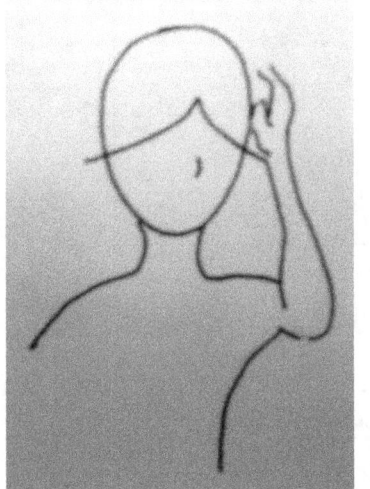

Rotation (turning head right and left)

Place hand on side of head. Your head should begin in the neutral position. Now attempt to turn head into the hand that has been placed on the side of your head. Push into hand for 2-3 seconds then relax. Repeat 2-4 times, and then do same procedure on the other side of your head.

As you must have noticed the resistive exercises encompass all the range of motions of your head and neck and likewise complete the extent of your strengthening. At this point it needs to be emphasized that all of the previous instructions are to be followed 'pain free'. The old adage 'no pain, no gain' is simply not true in this case. Pain causes damage to your tissues and will continue to irritate your neck and possibly increase your pain, which of course is not the intent. So as you move through each chapter the idea is to take it one step at a time going at your own pace. If there is constant pain present, then proceed very slowly attempting at no time to increase your level of pain. Sometimes just doing gentle range of motion will suffice to make a start. Once the pain has eased, and you are tolerating range of motion and can do without pain, then graduate to stretches and so forth. Others will be able to move more quickly and get to strengthening in no time at all, but once again nothing in this book that you do is to cause pain. If it does then your technique maybe wrong. You may be pushing yourself too far, and too fast, or you're simply not ready to move forward.

Chapter 7

Synergy…

I have found that often times it is better to have a synergistic model of health care. There are no magic bullets out there, and just like you, I wish there were. But let's work with what we have. We are always on the search for something better that we are not aware of. With chronic neck pain, as with anything else, there are no instant remedies that will fix the problem and let you go back to the time when pain was not an issue. The preceding chapters have helped you to identify things that you are doing that actually have caused you more pain. It is now within your control to minimize those effects and correct them by practicing and putting into practice what you have learned. This may not be easy for some of you, and in the beginning may even seem like it does not work. But given time, it will. Although you may not get rid of your pain 100 percent, you will be able to reduce it and hopefully to a point where your lifestyle is much improved. Pain is depressing and that depression can rob you of all that is good in your life. Now with the knowledge that you have gained through this program you have the ability to be proactive in your health and can act accordingly.

Neck pain sufferers have what is termed a chronic health condition, whatever the cause. Most chronic conditions worsen over time. Some reasons have all ready been stated. However, for some of us, the reasons are unknown, and we will continue to have flare ups. This simply means that for what ever reason our pain will return or increase for no apparent reason. The exercises and the strengthening you have learned to do will help considerably, but they are not a magic bullet! So sometimes it will be necessary to employ some other methods as well. In this chapter we will discuss those methods, and the benefit each one has and its effectiveness.

First of all let us discuss money. When you are ill, or even in chronic pain, money becomes an issue. Insurance often does not pick up the whole cost especially where alternative medicine is considered. However, the choice is still yours and what we discuss in this chapter are alternative methods, and are not for everyone. But it is your health and ultimately your choice as to whether the insurance company gets to dictate what you do or do not do regarding your health. There are many choices to be made and many opinions on those choices, it is all up to you.

Chiropractic

The primary emphasis on chiropractic care is the vertebrae of your spine. By their adjustments to the spine they restore the mobility of joints. In so doing it reduces the chronic irritation that occurs from a dysfunctional joint. This in turn reduces pain. Alignment also helps to restore more proper function to your nervous system due to the impact the dysfunctional joint has on the peripheral nerves that stem out from the spinal cord. Most chiropractors also have available in their offices modalities to help restore muscle function.

I have often found that when a person has in the past tried chiropractic care and has found it not to be beneficial they give up. It would be my suggestion that perhaps you try a different doctor. Just like in any profession there are many ways to do the job. Some MD's prefer Tylenol others prefer Ibuprofen; the same could be said of Chiropractors. At last count there were 112 different techniques that could be used to adjust the spine. Find one that works for you. Again let me state that this is not the magic bullet. One adjustment will not necessarily get you out of pain, but with regular care, just as in dentistry you will find that this is a good thing to do for your neck pain.

Acupuncture

Primary emphasis is on restoring the normal energy flow through out your body, thus allowing your body to heal. By the insertion of needles into key points along the meridian lines it is said to balance the energies and reduce any obstructions of flow. There are no nerve endings at these insertion points so the discomfort of the needle insertion is minimal. If you are finding that your health is deteriorating this may be a good thing to do as it can restore the electrical balance of your body and promote healing.

Massage

Primary emphasis is on muscles. The type of massage you need is called therapeutic. You do not need the "feel good stuff", it will not benefit your muscles as much. With chronic pain, you are often in spasms and will also have multiple trigger points. A massage therapist can help with these issues and make your muscles more workable and reduce the size of your trigger points. Massage therapy works well in conjunction with chiropractic care.

Supplements

A lot of chiropractors are familiar with nutritional supplementation and can give you advice on which is the best to take for your particular situation. We discussed supplementation in Chapter 2 as to which ones can be of benefit for pain. If it is your desire to go completely alternative, then one who is most familiar would be a Naturopath doctor. These doctors are trained in nutrition, herbal therapy, and supplementation. They can treat you for many other conditions beyond your pain, and will have more natural healing methods to prescribe.

This describes most of what is available here in the United States. Some other countries of course do things differently. The US is a little behind in alternative care, and at present, I understand, that there is a movement to take this choice away. You may find it wise to get on the band wagon to defend your right.

With that said, you most likely will find that from time to time these methods will also help to control the level of your pain, especially during periods of flare ups. Of course you will need to continue to practice your new moves and to become really proficient at adjusting your methods so that you minimize irritation to your neck. Always bear in mind the need to maintain center and to vary your activity so that you are constantly motioning in different ways to avoid static. As an example you will note that if someone sits beside you and you have to turn your head to talk to them this becomes uncomfortable in a short period of time. It is static and will need to be changed for you to avoid the discomfort and irritation. The most comfortable position is to be in your center - that center that was designed for you and no one else. In the last chapter you will find that I have summarized all of the key concepts and have put all of the exercises into one place. I did this for your benefit. After having studied this book you will be able to refer back to the last chapter to refresh your memory and to redefine your techniques.

As an added bonus I have also included some generalized back care tips. Much like brushing your teeth on a daily basis these practices will help to ensure that you keep a healthy spine.

Back Care Instructions

- **No reading in bed, no propping up on your elbows to read or supporting yourself with pillows to read**
- **Do not lay on the couch with your head propped up on the arm rest**
- **Use a pillow for your bed that will support your neck, any pillow that fits you will be sufficient as long as it supports your neck in neutral position**
- **When sleeping on your side use a pillow between your**

legs to keep the hips from tilting and only bend your knees to about 45 degrees, do not draw them up into your chest

- Never sleep on your stomach, bad for the low back
- Do not sit with your legs crossed except at the ankles and only if you can do this while staying on your sitting bones
- Sleep on a good firm mattress, not one with lumps and bumps or sags.

Chapter 8 –
Review of Key Concepts

The concepts in this book are very simple, very direct. Neck pain can be debilitating and interfere with even the simplest chores of daily living. Dependent on your own situation, this can seem hopeless. As a Chiropractor I have helped many people get relief from their pain, and have taught this program to each of them. Often they will come back to me and tell me how they are amazed that this works. They will tell me of a situation of when they had been in pain, did their shoulder shrugs and a couple of stretches, and it helped to relieve their pain. This of course does not happen instantly. You have to practice and be diligent about correcting your posture. Soon you will find that it is more uncomfortable to slouch then to sit up correctly! As a review this chapter goes over the concepts so that you can have a quick reference guide when you need to refresh your memory, or just to check and make sure you are on track.

Concept 1

It has been studied and found out that people who carry their head forward of their shoulders, carry hundreds of pounds of excess weight from gravitational forces. This produces stress on your neck, wear and tear and eventual pain, not to mention the use of energy and fatigue it produces.

Concept 2

Posture is important to help reduce fatigue and pain. Promoting your 'S' curve will help you to stay in your center and reduce the effect of gravity therefore reducing pain and irritation of your neck. The shoulder shrug will help you to find your correct posture, and the therapy ball will strengthen your core posture muscles.

Concept 3

Stretching exercise helps to relieve tired irritable muscles as well as to restore more proper motion of the muscles. The frog and scalenus muscle stretches will help you to achieve this. Do them slowly and gently, do not force the stretch.

Concept 4

Resistive exercises help to strengthen and tone the neck muscles. Using your hand as the resistive force makes this possible to do anywhere any time that is convenient simply by doing range of motion.

Concept 5

The scissor stance is imperative for widening your center and creating a strong balance. It reduces repetitive damage when used for bending and lifting by promoting the 'S' curve. It also reduces the amount of shirring force upon the spine.

Concept 6

Reducing the amount of repetitive stresses on your spine will reduce the amount of damage that occurs over time thus promoting a healthier spine over all and decreasing the amount of stress on muscles, ligaments and tendons. A proper posture, stance, bend, and lift help to reduce the forces of stress upon your body, therefore reducing your pain.

Exercises

Below is the scissor stance. This stance should be used for the majority of the time in conjunction with the shoulder shrug to find your proper posture.

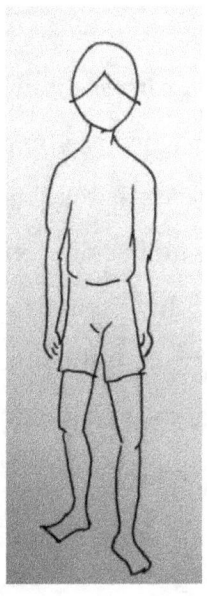

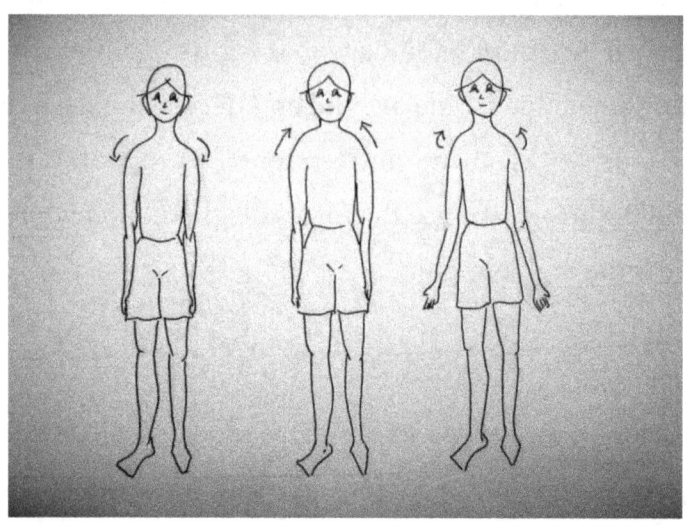

Shoulder Shrugs

Standing in front of a mirror looking straight into your eyes, roll your shoulders as far forward as you can, then raise your shoulders up towards your ears as high as they go. Now roll your shoulders back. When they go back far enough you will begin to feel them drop downwards. Let them drop in place but do not let them roll forward again. Check in the mirror to see that it looks right, it may not feel right but when looking at it you should be able to see your new and improved posture.

Therapy ball

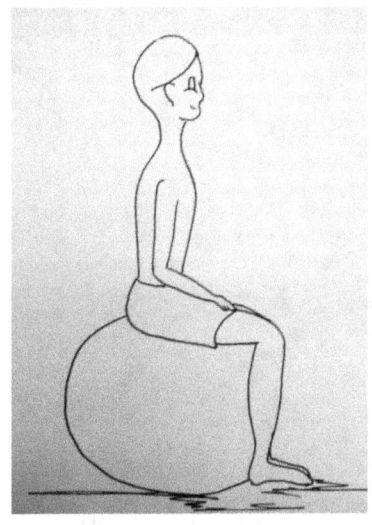

Remember the ball must be blown up big enough so that your thighs are parallel to the floor and feet can rest flat on the floor. Posture is centered by doing your shoulder shrugs. Arms are hanging down straight and bent at the elbow with hands resting on lap. Be careful not to let your arms move forward and round your shoulders.

Goal is to be able to sit for twenty minutes comfortably and without pain. Stop the exercise when you feel any discomfort and increase your time by one or two minutes the next day till eventually 20 minutes are achieved. Once the 20 minutes are accomplished you can do activity such as reading, or having dinner on the ball to pass the time.

Frog

With head in neutral stretch forward keeping head level and parallel to the floor. Stretch as far forward as comfortable, and then bring head backward till you feel the two muscles in the back of your neck stretch. Hold for the count of twenty then relax. Repeat 1 -2 times.

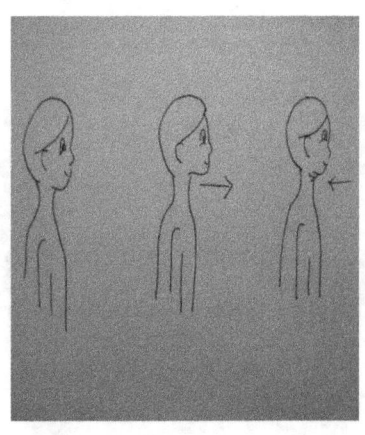

Scalenus stretches

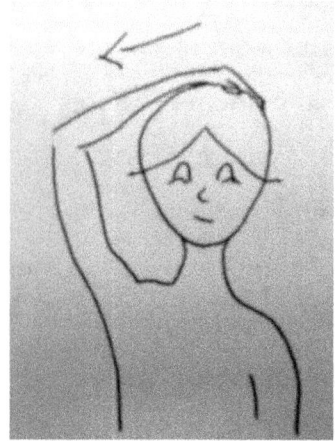

Looking straight ahead, take the pads of your fingers and gently pull your head towards your upheld arm.

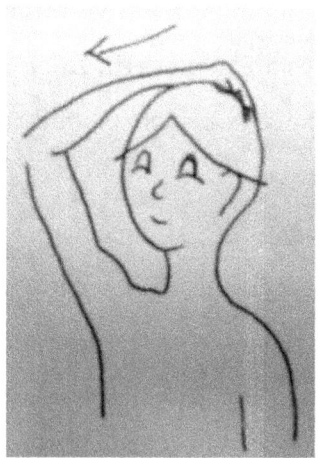

Turning your head toward your upheld arm, take the pads of your fingers and pull towards your same upheld arm

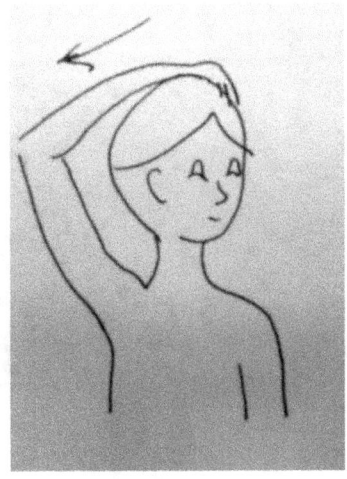

Now turn your head in the opposite direction, away from your upheld arm. Pulling with the pads of your fingers, pull your head towards the upheld arm.

Resistive exercises

Extension (bending head backward) Place your hand on the back of your head and push your head into your hand. Your hand should be around the crown of your head. Push the head into your hand then relax. Repeat this process 2-4 times. As an alternative

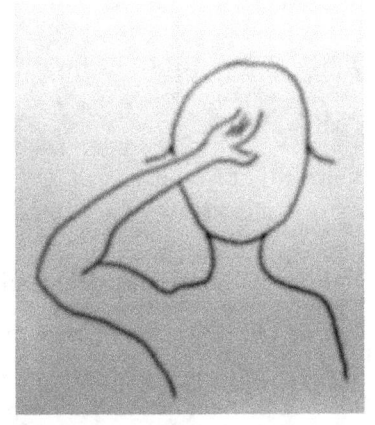

you can do this particular one against a wall by standing in center with your back as close to the wall as possible and instead of pushing into your hand, push into the wall.

Flexion (bending head forward)

With your head in neutral, place your hand on your forehead. Now push your head forward into your hand. Then relax your head after 2-3 seconds. Repeat 2-4 times to tolerance.

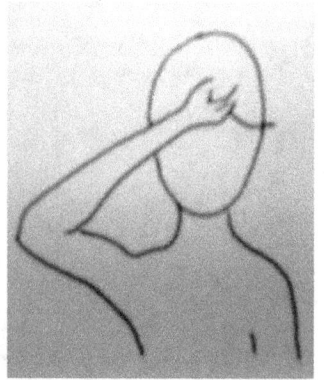

Lateral flexion (bending head sideways)

With head in neutral place, place hand on one side of the head. Now push head into hand for 2-3 seconds then relax. Repeat 2-4 times to tolerance. Do same procedure on the other side.

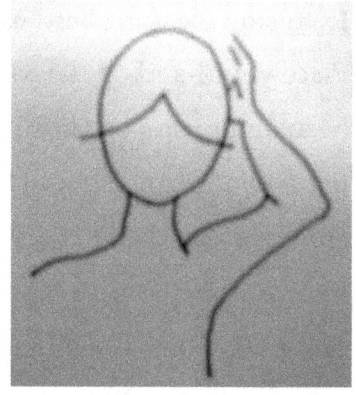

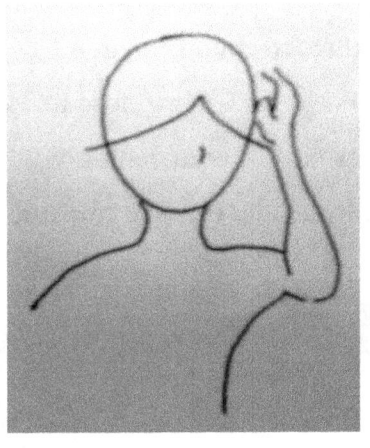

<u>Rotation</u> (turning head right and left) Place hand on side of head. Head is in neutral. Now attempt to turn head into the hand that has been placed on the side of your head. Push into hand for 2-3 seconds then relax. Repeat 2-4 times, and then do same procedure on the other side of your head.

Bending

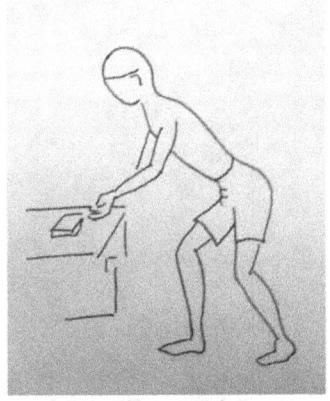

Notice that when using the scissor bend how the lower back is kept more straight and the knees are bent. You will also find that your neck does not flex as much either. This particular stance is more appropriate when bending or lifting.

Lifting

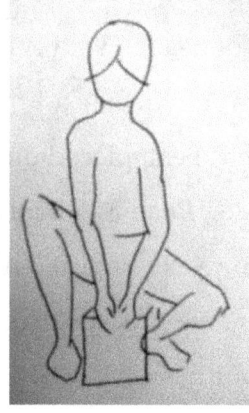

Note how close to the object you can get when picking up. Because you are close to the object it becomes part of your center, you also have more leverage and balance causing less stress and energy.

Torsion

Using the scissor stance, when twisting, helps to avoid the shearing force placed on the spine.

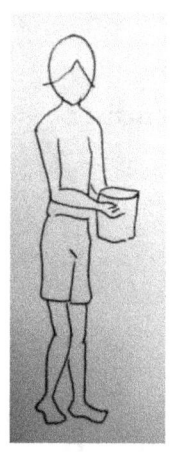

Go at your own pace and remember there is to be no pain with any of the exercises! Best wishes for you.

Dr. Judi Morris DC

References

Churchill Livingstone, Gray's Anatomy 38th edition, Skeletal system, Muscle, Nervous system

Gregory Plaugher, 1993 Textbook of Clinical Chiropractic, a specific biomechanical approach

Wikipedia Encylopedia, 2006 online source of meaning of pain

Medline Plus, 2006 Medical Encyclopedia – Arthritis

Journal of American Medical Association, 2003;289;2509-16

Balagot, R.C., Ehrenpreis, S., Greenberg, J. and Hyodo, M., "D-Phenylalanine in Human Chronic Pain", New York, Raven Press

Andrew Saul, PhD., Dr. Yourself

The Complete German Commission E Monographs, Therapeutic Guide to Herbal Medicines, Blumenthal, Busse, Goldberg, Gruenwald, Hall, Klein, Riggins & Rister